Primary Health Care in the Dental Office

Guest Editor

IRA B. LAMSTER, DDS, MMSc

DENTAL CLINICS OF NORTH AMERICA

www.dental.theclinics.com

October 2012 • Volume 56 • Number 4

SAUNDERS an imprint of ELSEVIER, Inc.

W.B. SAUNDERS COMPANY
A Division of Elsevier Inc.

1600 John F. Kennedy Boulevard • Suite 1800 • Philadelphia, Pennsylvania 19103-2899

http://www.dental.theclinics.com

DENTAL CLINICS OF NORTH AMERICA Volume 56, Number 4
October 2012 ISSN 0011-8532, ISBN 978-1-4557-4932-4

Editor: Yonah Korngold; y.korngold@elsevier.com

Dental Clinics of North America (ISSN 0011-8532) is published quarterly by Elsevier Inc., 360 Park Avenue South, New York, NY 10010-1710. Months of issue are January, April, July, and October. Business and Editorial Offices: 1600 John F. Kennedy Boulevard, Suite 1800, Philadelphia, PA 19103-2899. Periodicals postage paid at New York, NY and additional mailing offices. Subscription prices are $259.00 per year (domestic individuals), $447.00 per year (domestic institutions), $122.00 per year (domestic students/residents), $310.00 per year (Canadian individuals), $563.00 per year (Canadian institutions), $375.00 per year (international individuals), $563.00 per year (international institutions), and $184.00 per year (international and Canadian students/residents). International air speed delivery is included in all *Clinics* subscription prices. All prices are subject to change without notice. **POSTMASTER:** Send address changes to *Dental Clinics of North America*, Elsevier Health Sciences Division, Subscription Customer Service, 3251 Riverport Lane, Maryland Heights, MO 63043. **Customer Service (orders, claims, online, change of address): Elsevier Health Sciences Division, Subscription Customer Service, 3251 Riverport Lane, Maryland Heights, MO 63043. Tel: 1-800-654-2452 (U.S. and Canada). Fax: 314-447-8029. E-mail: journalscustomer service-usa@elsevier.com (for print support); journalsonlinesupport-usa@elsevier.com (for online support).**

Reprints. For copies of 100 or more, of articles in this publication, please contact the Commercial Reprints Department, Elsevier Inc., 360 Park Avenue South, New York, NY 10010-1710. Tel.: 212-633-3812; Fax: 212-462-1935; E-mail: reprints@elsevier.com.

The *Dental Clinics of North America* is covered in *MEDLINE/PubMed (Index Medicus), Current Contents/Clinical Medicine, ISI/BIOMED* and *Clinahl*.

Printed and bound by CPI Group (UK) Ltd, Croydon, CR0 4YY

Transferred to digital print 2012

Contributors

GUEST EDITOR

IRA B. LAMSTER, DDS, MMSc
Professor of Dental Medicine, Columbia University Mailman School of Public Health, Department of Health Policy & Management, Dean Emeritus, Columbia University College of Dental Medicine, New York, New York

AUTHORS

SHARON R. AKABAS, PhD
Associate Clinical Professor in Pediatrics, Director, MS in Nutrition Program, Institute of Human Nutrition, Columbia University Medical Center, New York, New York

DAVID ALBERT, DDS, MPH
Associate Professor of Dentistry, Section of Social and Behavioral Sciences, Director, Division of Community Health, Columbia University College of Dental Medicine, New York, New York

BONNIE R. BERNSTEIN, PhD
Adjunct Professor, Teachers College; Department of Pediatrics, Institute of Human Nutrition, Columbia University Medical Center, New York, New York

JOANNE D. CHOUINARD, DMD, MPH, MS
Department of Pediatrics, Institute of Human Nutrition, Columbia University Medical Center, New York, New York

HUGH DEVLIN, PhD, MSc, BSc, BDS
Professor Hugh Devlin, Professor of Restorative Dentistry, School of Dentistry, University of Manchester, Manchester, United Kingdom

AMANDA DEWUNDARA, BA
Columbia University College of Dental Medicine, New York, New York

CHESTER W. DOUGLASS, DMD, PhD
Professor, Department of Epidemiology, Harvard School of Public Health, Boston, Massachusetts

MICHAEL GLICK, DMD
William M. Feagans Professor, Dean, School of Dental Medicine, University at Buffalo, Buffalo, New York

J. MAX GOODSON, DDS, PhD
Senior Member of the Staff, Department of Applied Oral Sciences, The Forsyth Institute, Cambridge, Massachusetts

BARBARA L. GREENBERG, MSc, PhD
Acting Associate Dean of Research, Director, Institutional Research, Associate Professor, New Jersey Dental School, New Jersey

MONICA HALEM, MD
Clinical Assistant Professor, Department of Dermatology, Columbia University, New York, New York

JONATHAN HOGAN, MD
Professor of Medicine, Division of Nephrology, Department of Medicine, Columbia University Medical Center

CHANTÉ KARIMKHANI, BA, BA
3rd Year Medical Student, Columbia University College of Physicians and Surgeons, New York, New York

EVANTHIA LALLA, DDS, MS
Professor of Dental Medicine, Section of Oral and Diagnostic Sciences, Division of Periodontics, Columbia University College of Dental Medicine, New York, New York

IRA B. LAMSTER, DDS, MMSc
Professor of Dental Medicine, Columbia University Mailman School of Public Health, Department of Health Policy & Management, Dean Emeritus, Columbia University College of Dental Medicine, New York, New York

FOLARIN ODUSOLA, DDS
Associate Professor of Clinical Dental Medicine, Section of Adult Dentistry, Columbia University College of Dental Medicine, New York

JAI RADHAKRISHNAN, MD, MS, MRCP, FASN
Professor of Medicine, Division of Nephrology, Department of Medicine, Columbia University College of Physician and Surgeons, New York, New York

DAVID A. REZNIK, DDS
Chief, Dental Service, Grady Health System, Assistant Clinical Professor, Emory University School of Medicine, Atlanta, Georgia

JAYAPRIYAA SHANMUGHAM, BDS, MPH, DPH
Clinical Instructor, Department of Oral Health Policy and Epidemiology, Harvard School of Dental Medicine, Boston, Massachusetts

MARY TAVARES, DMD, MPH
Senior Clinical Investigator, Department of Applied Oral Sciences, The Forsyth Institute, Cambridge, Massachusetts; Harvard School of Dental Medicine, Boston, Massachusetts

ANGELA WARD, RDH, MA
Section of Social and Behavioral Sciences, Division of Community Health, Columbia University College of Dental Medicine, New York, New York

Contents

Preface ix

Ira B. Lamster

**Primary Care, the Dental Profession, and the Prevalence of Chronic Diseases
in the United States** 699

Chester W. Douglass and Jayapriyaa R. Shanmugham

> The population of the United States is aging rapidly, and the prevalence of
> chronic diseases will increase as the population grows and ages. The man-
> agement of chronic illnesses will become an increasing burden for primary
> care providers. This article suggests that dentists may need to monitor
> chronic disease and control the risk factors (ie, provide primary care) for
> their own dental patients.

The Assessment and Importance of Hypertension in the Dental Setting 731

Jonathan Hogan and Jai Radhakrishnan

> Many patients with hypertension have uncontrolled disease. The dental
> visit presents a unique opportunity to screen patients for undiagnosed
> and undertreated hypertension, which may lead to improved monitoring
> and treatment. Although there are no clinical studies, it is generally recom-
> mended that nonemergent procedures be avoided in patients with a blood
> pressure of greater than 180/110 mm Hg. Because of the high prevalence
> of disease and medication use for hypertension, dentists should be aware
> of the oral side effects of antihypertensive medications as well as the car-
> diovascular effects of medications commonly used during dental visits.

Tobacco Cessation in the Dental Office 747

David Albert and Angela Ward

> Evidence-based tobacco-cessation guidelines when used by clinicians
> are effective in reducing tobacco use and obtaining successful quits by
> patients. Dentists have been encouraged to provide instruction and inter-
> vention on tobacco cessation in the dental office. The dental provider is in
> the unique position to relate oral findings to the patient and to provide ad-
> vice to tobacco-using patients to quit. In addition, dentists are able to
> assess patients' self-addiction and level of readiness to quit tobacco
> use. With this information, dentists can assist in helping patients to stop
> using tobacco by providing appropriate pharmacotherapeutic aid and
> thus improve their oral and overall health.

Dermatology of the Head and Neck: Skin Cancer and Benign Skin Lesions 771

Monica Halem and Chanté Karimkhani

> Skin lesions are extremely common, and early detection of dangerous
> lesions makes skin cancer one of the most highly curable malignancies.
> By simply becoming aware of common lesions and their phenotypic

presentation, dental professionals are empowered to detect suspicious dermatologic lesions in unaware patients. This article serves as an introduction to skin cancer and benign skin lesions for dental professionals.

Nutrition and Physical Activity in Health Promotion and Disease Prevention: Potential Role for the Dental Profession   791

Sharon R. Akabas, Joanne D. Chouinard, and Bonnie R. Bernstein

Nutrition contributes to many of the leading causes of death in the United States, yet less than one-third of dental students feel competent to discuss the relationship of nutrition and systemic disease with their patients. The American Dental Association policy statements acknowledge a need for health professionals and organizations to provide continuing education to professionals and counseling to patients to combat the growing problems of overweight and obesity. Dentists can play a major role in educating patients to adopt a healthier lifestyle, including nutrition and physical activity recommendations. An understanding of the complexity of behavior change may enhance the dentist's ability to assist their patients in making desired changes.

Screening for Infectious Diseases in the Dental Setting   809

David A. Reznik

Human immunodeficiency virus (HIV) and hepatitis C virus (HCV) are 2 systemic infectious diseases that dental health care professionals can help identify with the goal of improving health outcomes, addressing health disparities, and improving the quality and quantity of life. Whether by identifying suspect oral lesions, as is the case with HIV infection, or offering rapid screening tests in the dental setting for both HIV and HCV, the dental team can play an important role in linkage to confirmatory diagnosis and care.

Assessment and Management of Patients with Diabetes Mellitus in the Dental Office   819

Evanthia Lalla and Ira B. Lamster

Diabetes mellitus is a serious chronic disease that affects many dental patients. Dental professionals have the potential and responsibility to assume an active role in the early identification, assessment, and management of their patients who present with or are at risk of developing diabetes. Close maintenance, meticulous monitoring of individual patient needs, and close collaboration with other health care professionals involved in the care will enable better control of the oral complications of diabetes and contribute to the better management of the patient's overall health status.

Obesity Prevention and Intervention in Dental Practice   831

Mary Tavares, Amanda Dewundara, and J. Max Goodson

Dentists have an important role in preventing and detecting oral and systemic diseases because of their diagnostic and screening abilities and the frequency of patient visits. These skills and practice paradigms should be considered in solving the obesity epidemic. The well-described connection between periodontal disease and diabetes is a reason for dentists to intervene in the rise of obesity. Dentists are in a unique position to identify and aid in treatment of obstructive sleep apnea, a condition associated with obesity and diabetes. Dentists can play a role in raising awareness of overweight status and obesity risk behaviors in children.

Identification of the Risk for Osteoporosis in Dental Patients   **847**

Hugh Devlin

This article describes how dentists can recognize osteoporosis before fractures develop, and discusses whether osteoporosis affects tooth loss or inhibits implant osseointegration. Some success in diagnosing osteoporosis has been obtained using clinical questionnaires that attempt to identify those who have strong risk factors for the disease, and analysis of the sparse trabeculation and thinning of the mandibular cortex often seen in dental panoramic radiographs. The role of osteoporosis in periodontal disease is unclear as there are many conflicting reports, but the evidence suggests that tooth loss may be more prevalent in patients with osteoporosis.

Assessing Systemic Disease Risk in a Dental Setting: A Public Health Perspective   **863**

Barbara L. Greenberg and Michael Glick

Screening and monitoring for systemic disease risk in a dental setting are valuable components for more effective disease prevention and control and health care delivery. This strategy can identify patients at increased risk of disease yet unaware of their increased risk and who may benefit from proven prevention/intervention strategies. The involvement of oral health care professionals in strategies to identify individuals at risk for coronary heart disease and diabetes will extend preventive and screening efforts necessary to slow the development of these diseases, and provide a portal for individuals who do not see a physician on a regular basis to enter into the general health care system.

Concluding Remarks   **875**

Ira B. Lamster and Folarin Odusola

Index   **879**

DENTAL CLINICS OF NORTH AMERICA

FORTHCOMING ISSUES

January 2013
Pediatric Dentistry
Joel H. Berg, DDS, MS, *Guest Editor*

April 2013
Evidence-based Women's Oral Health
Leslie Halpern, MD, DDS, PhD, MPH, and
Linda Kaste, DDS, MS, PhD, *Guest Editors*

RECENT ISSUES

July 2012
Regenerative Endodontics
Sami M.A. Chogle, BDS, DMD, MSD, and
Harold E. Goodis, DDS, *Guest Editors*

April 2012
Sleep Medicine and Dentistry
Ronald Attanasio, DDS, MSEd, MS, and
Dennis R. Bailey, DDS, *Guest Editors*

January 2012
Oral Surgery for the General Dentist
Harry Dym, DDS, and Orrett E. Ogle, DDS,
Guest Editors

RELATED INTEREST

Primary Care: Clinics in Office Practice
June 2012 (Volume 39, No. 2)
Chronic Disease Management
Brooke Salzman, MD, Lauren Collins, MD, and Emily R. Hajjar, PharmD,
Guest Editors

Preface

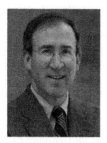

Ira B. Lamster, DDS, MMSc
Guest Editor

As the population of the United States expands, ages, and becomes more diverse, a greater number of people will be living with chronic diseases. These disorders will be managed over decades, and millions of individuals will use multiple medications to treat conditions such as hypertension, diabetes mellitus, cardiovascular diseases, respiratory diseases, and infectious diseases. Management of these disorders is a challenge for the health care system and for affected individuals. With the recognized shortage of primary health care providers, new opportunities and possibilities for managing chronic diseases must be identified. As it assesses its future, the dental profession must consider what part it will play in caring for the health, not just the oral health, of patients seen in dental offices.

Dental care has advanced dramatically in the past decades. Older adults in the United States now routinely retain teeth for a lifetime, and procedures and techniques are available to restore even the most compromised dentition. Patients requiring extensive restorative services are often older and must be evaluated for the effect of oral disease on their general health as well as for their ability to tolerate multiple visits required for complex oral rehabilitation. There are many examples. Patients with poorly controlled diabetes mellitus will present with a greater extent and severity of periodontal disease and may also be affected by dry mouth and *Candida* infection. If patients with diabetes are metabolically well-controlled, they may experience hypoglycemic episodes in the dental office. The patient with a cardiovascular disorder requiring anticoagulation therapy must be carefully managed if oral surgical procedures are planned. Further, it is critically important to maintain a functional masticatory system throughout one's lifetime. Poor oral function, and compromised masticatory function, has been shown to be associated with the development of the frailty syndrome in the elderly.[1]

Data on visits to oral health care providers argue for dental professionals to be more involved in the assessment of the health of their patients. Almost 70% of adults visited a dental professional in the last year for which data is available (2010).[2] Further, there is a portion of the population that sees a dental provider, but not a medical provider. Data from the US Medical Expenditure Panel Survey indicated that about a quarter of the US population did not see a medical provider in the last year for which data is available (2008), but 37% of these children and 23% of these adults visited a dental provider.[3]

Dent Clin N Am 56 (2012) ix–xi
http://dx.doi.org/10.1016/j.cden.2012.07.001
0011-8532/12/$ – see front matter

The larger issue of defining a primary health care provider is germane to this discussion. The American Academy of Family Practitioners defines primary care as including "health promotion, disease prevention, health maintenance, counseling, patient education, diagnosis, and treatment of acute and chronic illnesses in a variety of health care settings (eg, office, inpatient, critical care, long-term care, home care, day care, etc)."[4] While not mentioning dental offices, this broad definition is well aligned with the core values and beliefs of the dental profession and is synergistic with what is considered appropriate dental care.

This monograph reviews some of the most obvious activities that are, or could be, part of a more comprehensive management of patients seen in the dental office. A number of these activities, including evaluation of hypertension by dentists, have been discussed for decades.[5] Others, such as assessment of risk for diabetes mellitus, have been shown in a recent prospective study of patients seen in the dental clinic to yield a larger than expected number of patients who would be classified as having diabetes mellitus, and an even greater number who would qualify as "prediabetic."[6] The opportunity for early intervention, with referral to the appropriate provider for medical care, represents an unrealized health care opportunity. Other articles address the identification of individuals with infectious diseases, and the dental professions' role in smoking cessation. Use of oral fluid-based testing for infection with the human immunodeficiency virus (HIV) in the dental setting has also been suggested for some time[7] and can be expanded to include identification of hepatitis C infection. Involvement of the dental profession in smoking cessation activities is supported by the development of a model program in a dental school setting.[8] In both cases, the oral cavity figures prominently in the clinical presentation of disease. Oral lesions are common in HIV infection, including the appearance of distinct lesions,[9] and smoking and total exposure to cigarettes are primary risk factors for both periodontal disease[10] and oral squamous cell carcinoma.[11]

Articles also cover other relevant activities that can be adopted by dental professionals. Considering the percentage of the US population that visits the dentist in a year, even a modest change of behavior as a result of this new practice paradigm can have a very beneficial effect on the health of the nation.

This issue of the *Dental Clinics of North America* brings the general concept of primary care health activity in the dental office together in one volume. Other topics could have been included and likely will be added to the discussion if this activity becomes a more prominent part of dental practice.

Ira B. Lamster, DDS, MMSc
Columbia University Mailman School of Public Health
Department of Health Policy & Management
Dean Emeritus
Columbia University College of Dental Medicine
722 West 168th Street
New York, NY 10032

E-mail address:
ibl1@columbia.edu

REFERENCES

1. Semba RD, Blaum CS, Bartali B, et al. Denture use, malnutrition, frailty, and mortality among older women living in the community. J Nutr Health Aging 2006;10(2):161–7.

2. Centers for Disease Control and Prevention (CDC). Behavioral Risk Factor Surveillance System Survey Data. Visited the dentist or dental clinic within the past year for any reason. Nationwide (States and DC). Atlanta (GA): US Department of Health and Human Services, Centers for Disease Control and Prevention; 2010.
3. Strauss SM, Alfano MC, Shelley D, et al. Identifying unaddressed systemic health conditions at dental visits: patients who visited dental practices but not general health care providers in 2008. Am J Public Health 2012;102(2):253–5.
4. AAFP website. Available at: http://www.aafp.org/online/en/home/policy/polices/p/primarycare.printerview.html. Definition #1–-Primary Care. Accessed April 9, 2012.
5. Welborn JF. Routine screening for hypertension in dental practice: fundamental discipline of dental education. J Dent Ed 1973;37(11):38–40.
6. Lalla E, Kunzel C, Burkett S, et al. Identification of unrecognized diabetes and pre-diabetes in a dental setting. J Dent Res 2011;90(7):855–60.
7. Glick M. Rapid HIV testing in the dental setting. J Am Dent Assoc 2005;136(9): 1206, 1208.
8. Seidman DF, Albert D, Singer SR, et al. Serving underserved and hard-core smokers in a dental school setting. J Dent Ed 2002;66(4):507–13.
9. Bodhade AS, Ganvir SM, Hazarey VK. Oral manifestations of HIV infection and their correlation with CD4 count. J Oral Sci 2011;53(2):203–11.
10. Kinane DF, Chestnutt IG. Smoking and periodontal disease. Crit Rev Oral Biol Med 2000;11(3):356–65.
11. Blot WJ, McLaughlin JK, Winn DM, et al. Smoking and drinking in relation to oral and pharyngeal cancer. Cancer Res 1988;48(11):3282–7.

Primary Care, the Dental Profession, and the Prevalence of Chronic Diseases in the United States

Chester W. Douglass, DMD, PhD[a],*,
Jayapriyaa R. Shanmugham, BDS, MPH, DPH[b]

KEYWORDS

- Chronic disease • Primary care • Aging population • Disease burden

KEY POINTS

- Chronic diseases are the major causes of death among adults in the United States.
- Chronic disease prevalence increases with age.
- The United States population is aging rapidly.
- The prevalence of chronic diseases will increase as the population grows and ages.
- The management of chronic illnesses will become an increasing burden for primary care providers.
- Dentists may need to monitor chronic disease and control the risk factors (ie, provide primary care) for their own dental patients.

PRIMARY CARE

Primary care is the principal point of consultation for patients within a health care system, usually an MD who is a general practitioner or family physician. Increasingly, however, nurse practitioners, physician assistants, or pharmacists are serving as primary care providers. Patients are then referred for secondary specialty care or tertiary subspecialty care. The role of the primary care provider is to monitor patients' health, and assess and control risk factors for acute and chronic disease.

Because the majority of the United States population has seen a dentist in the past 24 months, and as dentists must increasingly monitor the chronic disease problems of their dental patients, there is a proposal that dentists could and should serve as the primary care provider for their dental patients. This article documents the epidemiology of chronic disease in the United States and sets the stage for a discussion of

[a] Department of Epidemiology, Harvard School of Public Health, 677 Huntington Avenue, Boston, Massachusetts; [b] Department of Oral Health Policy and Epidemiology, Harvard School of Dental Medicine, 188 Longwood Avenue, Boston, Massachusetts
* Corresponding author.
E-mail address: chester_douglass@hsdm.harvard.edu

Dent Clin N Am 56 (2012) 699–730
http://dx.doi.org/10.1016/j.cden.2012.07.002
0011-8532/12/$ – see front matter © 2012 Published by Elsevier Inc.

dental.theclinics.com

the role that dentists can serve as primary care providers, at least for their own dental patients.

AGING OF THE POPULATION

Chronic diseases increase with increasing age. In the United States the number of adults aged 65 years and older has been dramatically increasing over the past 30 years.[1,2] The annual population growth rate from 1950 to 2006 was 1.2% with the total population increasing from 151 million up to 299 million.[3] During this period, the population of adults aged 65 to 74 years grew substantially from 8 million to 19 million persons. Those 75 years and older grew fastest, from 4 million to 18 million persons. Overall the total population increased by 9.7% (281.4–308.7 million) from 2000 to 2010 while the older population (65 years and older) increased by 15.1% (35–40.3 million). By the year 2029 it is predicted that all baby boomers (born in the 1946–1964 time period) will be 65 years and older, representing to 10% of the entire population in 2030 (**Figs. 1–5**).[4]

CHRONIC DISEASE IN THE UNITED STATES

In the United States, chronic conditions have significantly affected the nation at the social, individual, and economic levels. Consider the following facts about chronic disease in the United States:

- Each year 7 out of 10 deaths are caused by chronic diseases.[5]
- In 2005 1 out of every 2 adults older than 21 had at least one chronic illness.[6]
- About 25% of those with chronic illness have one or more daily activity limitations.
- Nearly 75% of all the health care expenses in the United States are spent on those with chronic conditions.
- In 2006 the annual health care expenditure was more than $7000 per person, which is 3 times the amount spent in 1990.[7]

The most common chronic conditions that cause significant morbidity, mortality, and economic impact are heart disease, diabetes, stroke, cancer, asthma, obesity, and oral diseases. All of these chronic conditions are preventable, and the burden

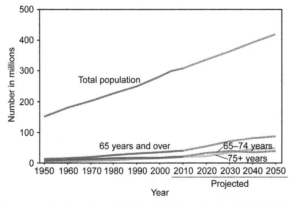

Fig. 1. Population growth. (*Data from* National Center for Health Statistics, United States, 2008. Population data from U.S. Census Bureau.)

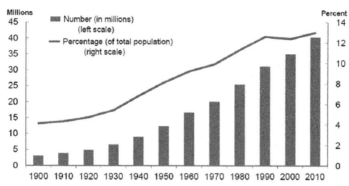

Fig. 2. Population 65 years and older by size and percentage of total population: 1900 to 2010. (*Data from* US Census Bureau, decennial census of population, 1900 to 2010. 2010 Census Summary File 1.)

of these chronic diseases can be lessened by improved health care and, most importantly, prevention and early diagnosis.

CURRENT TRENDS

The most common preventable chronic diseases are the leading causes of death and disability in the United States.[8] Heart disease, cancer, and stroke account for the major causes of death among adults aged 25 years and older.[9] Whereas cancer was the leading cause of death for those younger than 65 years, heart disease was the leading cause of death among those older than 65. The ranking of these 3 leading causes of death (heart disease, cancer, and stroke) did not change from 1980 to 2007. In 2005, 133 million Americans—almost 1 out of every 2 adults—had at least one chronic illness, which is expected to increase to 171 million persons with chronic diseases in 2030.[10] Exacerbating the burden of chronic illness is the fact that about one-fourth of people with chronic conditions have one or more limitations of daily activity.[6] Hence, treatment of chronic disease requires the additional expense for support needed to carry out the daily activities of living. By 2003 the economic burden of chronic disease had risen to $277 billion.[11] De Vol and Bedroussian[11] calculated that with continuation of similar trends the projected costs for 2023 would be $790 billion, a nearly 3-fold increase in 20 years.

Age Group	Percent Change 2000 to 2010
65 to 69	30.4
70 to 74	4.7
75 to 79	-1.3
80 to 84	16.1
85 to 89	29.8
90 to 95	30.2
95 to 99	25.9
100+	5.8

Fig. 3. Percent change in US population by age group: 2000 to 2010. (*Data from* US Census Bureau decennial census of population, 1900–2010.)

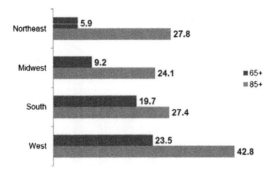

Fig. 4. Percent change by selected older age group by region: 2000 to 2010. (*Data from* 2010 Census, US Census Bureau; Census 2000.)

However, this huge increase in health care costs does not need to occur. With prevention, health education, and better primary health care the United States could achieve significant savings. In 2000, approximately 61 million people (21% of the population) had multiple chronic conditions.[12] Those with 5 or more chronic conditions report on average up to 15 physician visits and fill more than 50 prescriptions in a year. Among children the rates of chronic diseases such as asthma, obesity, and behavior and learning problems have increased from 12.8% in 1994 to 26.6% in 2006.[13] This trend is alarming because as the younger generations age through their life span, these chronic conditions are likely to emerge as major health problems for millions of middle-aged adults. The most prevalent primary disease problems are explored here to assess the extent of the current disease burden and trends for the future.

Heart Disease

At present in the United States, heart disease is the leading cause of death. Pharmaceuticals and risk-factor control have turned heart disease into a chronic disease process, resulting, ironically, in high and rising costs of medical care. In 2010 the American Heart Association (AHA) estimated the economic burden of cardiovascular disease (CVD) in 2010 to be $316.4 billion.[14] In 2009 a report by the National Center for Health Statistics (NCHS) observed an overall decline in the number of deaths due to heart disease.[9] However, it remains the leading cause of death among adults aged 65 years and older (**Fig. 6**). According to a report by the AHA based on data from the National Health and Nutrition Examination Survey (NHANES), National Heart,

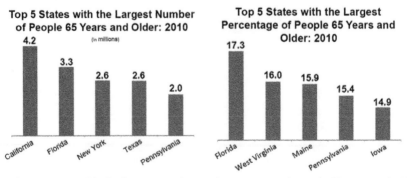

Fig. 5. Top 5 states with the largest number and percentage of people 65 years and older: 2010. (*Data from* 2010 Census, US Census Bureau.)

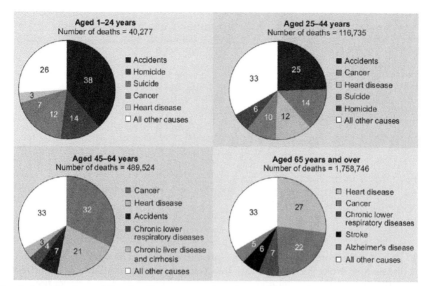

Fig. 6. Distribution of five leading causes of death in the US, by age group: Preliminary NCHS data, 2009. (*From* Miniño AM. Death in the United States, 2009. NCHS data brief, no 64. Hyattsville, MD: National Center for Health Statistics, 2011.)

Lung, and Blood Institute (NHLBI), and the NCHS, 36.2% of adults aged 20 years and older were diagnosed with CVD in 2008.[15] Of all deaths reported in 2006, about 26% (more than 1 in every 4 deaths) were caused by heart disease.[16] The death rate caused by CVD in 2005 to 2007 was 262.7 per 100, 000 and the financial burden in 2007 was approximately $287 billion, which included both direct and indirect costs (indirect costs are from loss of productivity/mortality). In 2003 the Centers for Disease Control and Prevention (CDC) reported that approximately 37% of adults had 2 or more CVD risk factors such as high blood pressure, high cholesterol, diabetes, smoking, inactivity, and obesity.[17] Probably primarily because of pharmaceutical use, since 1960 the percentage of adults with high cholesterol has decreased by almost half.[3] Data from the National Health Interview Survey (NHIS) conducted by NCHS, CDC, show a slight decline in the prevalence of heart disease in recent years; however, it still remains high among adults aged 65 years and older (**Figs. 7** and **8**).[18] Better treatment

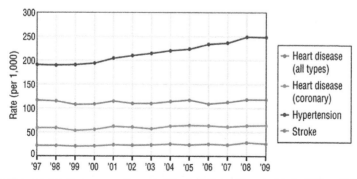

Fig. 7. Cardiovascular disease prevalence in US adults (age 18 and older). 1997 to 2009. * Rates presented are crude rates. (*From* U.S. Environmental Protection Agency (EPA). (2008) EPA's 2008 Report on the Environment. National Center for Environmental Assessment, Washington, DC; EPA/600/R-07/045F. Available from the National Technical Information Service, Springfield, VA, and online at http://www.epa.gov/roe.)

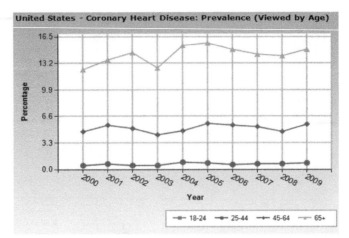

Fig. 8. United States coronary heart disease: prevalence (viewed by age). (*From* Division for Heart Disease and Stroke Prevention: Data Trends & Maps Web site. Atlanta (GA): US Department of Health and Human Services, Centers for Disease Control and Prevention (CDC), National Center for Chronic Disease Prevention and Health Promotion; 2010. Available at: http://www.cdc.gov/dhdsp/.)

procedures, increased awareness of health, and greater control of risk factors have contributed to the decline. However, with the increase in the aging population the economic burden from heart disease will remain very high.

Cancer

Owing to earlier diagnosis, earlier treatment methods, and greater control of risk factors, living with cancer has become a chronic condition. According to data from the Surveillance, Epidemiology and End Results (SEER) database of the National Cancer Institute (NCI), currently the overall estimated prevalence in the United States for all types of cancer is 12 million (4% of the United States population) (**Fig. 9**).[19] Of the survivors approximately 60% are 65 years and older, as these survivors were diagnosed more than 20 years ago. The prevalence of cancer has been steadily increasing

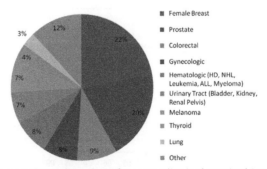

Fig. 9. Types of cancer estimated number of persons alive in the United States diagnosed with cancer on January 1, 2008 by site (N = 11.9 million). (*Data from* Howlader N, Noone AM, Krapcho M, et al. SEER cancer statistics review, 1975–2008. Bethesda (MD): National Cancer Institute; 2011. Available at: http://seer.cancer.gov/csr/1975_2008/, based on November 2010 SEER data submission, posted to the SEER Web site, 2011.)

over the years and remains the second leading cause of death in the United States.[5] In 2011 approximately 572,000 deaths were attributable to cancer as estimated by the American Cancer Society (ACS).[20] In 2009, overall 8% of adults aged 18 years and older reported a previous diagnosis of cancer.[21] The vast majority of cancer patients live with the disease (**Fig. 10**). Based on SEER data from 2004 to 2008, the death rates were only 9.0% between 45 and 54 years of age; 18.0% between 55 and 64 years; 24.8% between 65 and 74 years; and 29.3% between 75 and 84 years.[19]

Lung cancer is the leading cause of death from cancer among men and women.[22] More than 80% of lung cancers are due to smoking or exposure to second-hand smoking.[23] However, the most common types of cancers overall are breast (22%), prostate (20%), and colorectal (9%). Among men the most common types of cancers in 2007 included cancers of the prostrate, lung, and colon and rectum.[20] For women the most common types diagnosed in 2007 were breast, lung, and colon/rectal cancers (**Figs. 11** and **12**).

Stroke

Stroke is the third most common cause of death in the United States.[24] More than 1 million adults are disabled from stroke, most of whom are unable to perform simple daily tasks. Among adults aged 18 years and older the prevalence of stroke has remained steady over the years (see **Figs. 7** and **8**). Data from BRFSS show no change in the overall median percentage of adults with a history of stroke, with 2.5% in 2005 to 2.6% in 2010 (**Fig. 13**).[25] The prevalence of stroke is higher with increasing age: 8.5% of respondents aged 65 years and older reported a history of stroke in 2009 (**Table 1**). According to NHANES and NCHS data from 2005 to 2008, 7 million Americans aged 20 years and older reported being diagnosed with stroke.[15] Mortality data from 2007 indicate that stroke accounted for about 1 of every 18 deaths in the United States. From 1997 to 2007, the death rate attributable to stroke fell 34.3%, and the actual number of stroke deaths declined by 18.8%. As with heart disease, the financial burden of stroke is significant, with estimated costs up to $62.7 billion in 2007.[24]

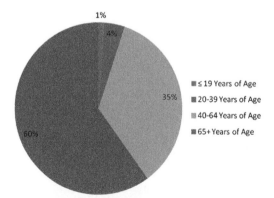

Fig. 10. Estimated number of persons alive in the United States diagnosed with cancer on January 1, 2008 by current age (invasive/first primary cases only, N = 11.9 million survivors). (*Data from* Howlader N, Noone AM, Krapcho M, et al. SEER cancer statistics review, 1975–2008. Bethesda (MD): National Cancer Institute. Available at: http://seer.cancer.gov/csr/1975_2008/, based on November 2010 SEER data submission, posted to the SEER Web site, 2011; and Altekruse S, Kosary C, Krapcho M, et al. SEER cancer statistics review, 1975–2008. Bethesda (MD): National Cancer Institute; 2011. Available at: http://seer.cancer.gov/csr/1975_2008/.)

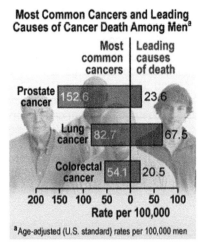

Fig. 11. Most common cancers and leading causes of cancer death among men. Age-adjusted (US standard) rates per 100,000 men. (*From* Centers for Disease Control and Prevention. Cancer statistics. Available at: http://www.cdc.gov/Features/dsCancerStatistics/.)

Diabetes

Diabetes mellitus has been increasing in incidence in the United States over the past 20 years (**Fig. 14**).[26] Of greater concern is that the prevalence of diabetes is predicted to increase further in the next 16 years (**Table 2**). Diabetes is the seventh leading cause of death in the United States.[27] It continues to be leading cause of kidney failure, leg amputations, and blindness among adults aged 20 to 74 years.[28] Diabetes is also a major contributor to heart disease and stroke.[27] According to the National Diabetes Surveillance System (NDSS), currently 26 million people in the United States are affected by diabetes. In 2010 approximately 10.9 million adults 65 years and older and 1.9 million adults 20 years and older had diabetes. A survey by NHANES reported

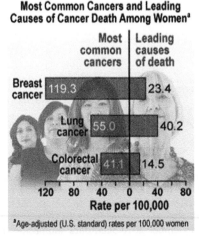

Fig. 12. Most common cancers and leading causes of cancer death among women. Age-adjusted (US standard) rates per 100,000 women. (*From* Centers for Disease Control and Prevention. Cancer statistics. Available at: http://www.cdc.gov/Features/dsCancerStatistics/.)

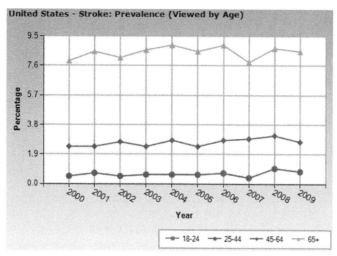

Fig. 13. Prevalence of stroke in the US by age: 2000–2009. (*From* Division for Heart Disease and Stroke Prevention. Data trends & maps Web site. Atlanta (GA): US Department of Health and Human Services, Centers for Disease Control and Prevention (CDC), National Center for Chronic Disease Prevention and Health Promotion; 2010. Available at: http://www.cdc.gov/dhdsp/.)

that between 2005 and 2008, 26.9% of all adults aged 20 years or older had diagnosed or undiagnosed diabetes. In 2005 to 2008, based on fasting glucose or hemoglobin A_{1c} levels, it was reported that 35% of adults aged 20 years and older had prediabetes. According to the BRFSS an upward trend was observed in the median percentage of people reported to have diabetes from 2004 to 2010.[25] Among all age groups the percentage of the United States population diagnosed with diabetes has been increasing since 1980, with the highest increase among 65- to 74-year-olds.[28] The financial burden from diabetes and diabetes-related complications is high and has been increasing over the years.[29] The annual cost for treating a person with diabetes is 5 times more than for a person without diabetes. The cost of diabetes increased from $132 billion in 2002 to $174 billion in 2007. By 2025 an estimated cost of $350 billion is predicted, making diabetes an increasingly serious chronic disease problem.

Asthma

Asthma is a chronic respiratory disorder that affects all age groups in the United States. At present, 18.7 million adults and 7 million children have asthma.[22] Children,

Table 1				
Prevalence percent of stroke among US adults 18 years and above (2000, 2009)				
Age Groups Year	**18–24 years Percentage (95% CI)**	**25–44 years Percentage (95% CI)**	**45–64 years Percentage (95% CI)**	**65 + years Percentage (95% CI)**
2000	—	0.5 (0.3–0.8)	2.4 (2.0–2.8)	7.9 (7.2–8.7)
2009	—	0.8 (0.6–1.0)	2.7 (2.3–3.1)	8.5 (7.6–9.4)

Abbreviation: CI, confidence interval.
  Data from National Health Interview Survey (NHIS), National Center for Health Statistics (NCHS), CDC.

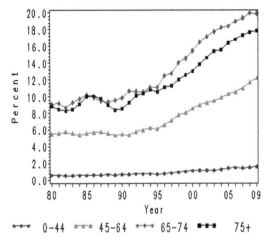

Fig. 14. Percentage of civilian, noninstitutionalized population with diabetes in the United States, 1980 to 2009. (*Data from* NHANES.)

women, African Americans, and those below the federal poverty level have the highest prevalence of asthma.[30] According to data from the 2001 to 2009 National Health Interview Surveys among persons of all ages, the prevalence of asthma increased from 7.3% (20.3 million) in 2001 to 8.2% (24.6 million) in 2009, a 12.3% increase (**Fig. 15**). Among children (0–17 years) the prevalence was 9.6% in 2009. Data from BRFSS show a similar trend whereby the median percentage of people who reported current asthma increased from 7.3% in 2000 to 9.0% in 2010.[25] The data also reported an increase in lifetime asthma prevalence from 10.6% (median percent) in 2000 to 13.8% in 2010 (**Fig. 16**).

The health costs from asthma are high, and the financial burden continues to increase. Health care expenses for asthma increased to $3259 per person from 2002 to 2007. Total asthma-associated medical expenditure increased from $48.6 billion in 2002 to $50.1 billion in 2007. The costs are not only financial but also in lost productivity. In 2008 more than 59% of children and 33% of adults missed school or work because of asthma.

Table 2
Prevalence of diabetes among United States adults (age 18+ years) (Percentage)

Year	18–24 years Percentage (95% CI)	25–44 years Percentage (95% CI)	45–64 years Percentage (95% CI)	65+ years Percentage (95% CI)
1999–2000	—	4.5 (2.9–7.0)	12.9 (9.9–16.6)	16.5 (11.4–23.3)
2001–2002	—	5.6 (4.1–7.7)	12.7 (9.4–16.9)	24.2 (20.2–28.9)
2003–2004	1.6 (0.9–2.6)	4.3 (2.6–7.1)	14.3 (11.1–18.4)	25.4 (19.3–32.6)
2005–2006	—	5.3 (3.7–7.5)	13.2 (10.1–17.1)	25.3 (20.6–30.5)
2007–2008	—	4.2 (2.8–6.2)	15.4 (12.4–18.9)	29.9 (26.5–33.5)

Data from NHANES (The National Health and Nutrition Examination Survey), National Center for Health Statistics, CDC.

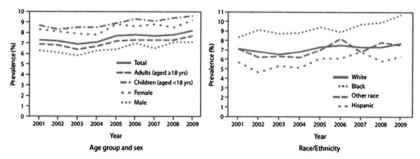

Fig. 15. Prevalence of asthma by year, age, race, and gender. (*From* Centers for Disease Control and Prevention (CDC). Vital signs: asthma prevalence, disease characteristics, and self-management education: United States, 2001–2009. MMWR Morb Mortal Wkly Rep 2011;60(17):547–52.)

Obesity

Obesity is defined as a high body weight that is considered unhealthy for a given height, which can be determined using the body mass index (BMI). The BMI is a composite measure of overall body fat distribution and is calculated by dividing weight in kilograms (kg) by the square of height in meters (m²).[31] Adults with a BMI of 30 or higher are considered obese. Obesity prevalence has been increasing since the 1970s and the rates continue to rise.[32] Alarming data from the NHANES now show that one-third of United States adults (33.8%) are obese. Among children and adolescents aged 2 to 19 years, 12.5 million are obese (17%). Since 1985 obesity in this age group has increased significantly across the country, with rates rising to about 30% in several states (**Fig. 17**).[33] Obesity significantly increases the risk for several chronic conditions including heart disease, diabetes, cancer (endometrial, breast, and colon), hypertension, stroke, liver disease, arthritis, and infertility.[34] Overweight (but not obese), which is defined by a BMI of 25 and higher, is also a significant risk factor for several chronic conditions. The costs of the medical care of obesity in the United States are very high, with estimated in 2008 at $147 billion.[35] The economic impact from obesity costs is significant, owing to the direct and indirect costs associated with overweight and obesity.[36,37] Direct costs for obesity include diagnostic and treatment costs. Indirect costs include income lost from decreased productivity, restricted activity, absenteeism, and loss of future income by premature death. Obesity is a major national health problem that in the future will contribute toward the increasing rates of chronic disease.

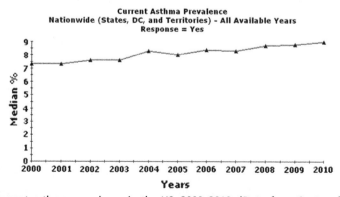

Fig. 16. Current asthma prevalence in the US: 2000–2010. (*Data from* Centers for Disease Control and Prevention Behavioral Risk Factor Surveillance System.)

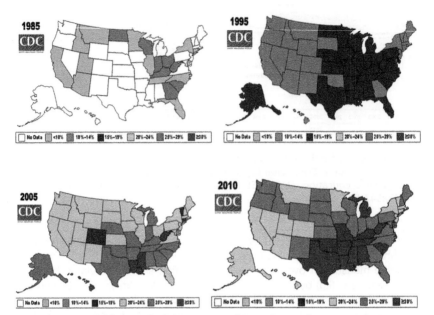

Fig. 17. Obesity in children and adolescents aged 2 to 19 years by state and year.

Oral Disease

Oral diseases are the most prevalent chronic conditions in the United States population. Patients with both chronic diseases and oral diseases will increasingly be seen in the dental office. Chronic oral conditions such as dental caries, periodontal disease, and oral cancer cause pain and disability and incur high treatment costs. In the United States more than 90% of adults aged 20 to 64 years have dental caries.[38] Dental caries is the most common preventable chronic illness among children.[39] Children living in the lower socioeconomic areas are at higher risk for dental caries and for not having it treated. Dental caries can be painful, and thus affects the quality of life among children through, for example, school absenteeism, difficulty eating, and difficulty swallowing.[40] Whereas percentages of untreated cavities have declined from 1971 to 1974 (25.0% in children aged 2–5 and 54.7% in children aged 6–19 years), data for the most recent time period (2001–2004) still show high levels of untreated cavities: 19.5% in children aged 2 to 5 and 22.9% in children aged 6 to 19 (**Fig. 18**).[39] The long-term effects of dental caries include high and rising need for dental care in older adults and the elderly.

Periodontitis is characterized by the loss of the attachment tissue and bone that support the teeth.[41] Severe periodontal disease eventually results in tooth loss. Among adults, periodontitis is a leading cause of bleeding, pain, infection, loose teeth, and tooth loss. Approximately 75% of adults in the United States are affected by some form of periodontitis (gingivitis or periodontitis). The prevalence of periodontal disease is highest among those 50 to 64 years old. In 2008, data from BRFSS reported 43.1% of adults aged 65 years or older having lost 6 or more teeth because of caries or periodontal disease. Overall, the prevalence of periodontitis has decreased since the late 1990s.[42] However, recent research findings have observed a positive association between periodontal disease and major chronic conditions such as heart disease and diabetes.[43] The incidence of periodontal disease will probably increase in many older adults as they continue to retain more of their natural dentition.

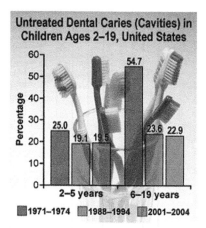

Fig. 18. Untreated dental caries (cavities) in children aged 2 to 19 years, United States. (*From* Centers for Disease Control and Prevention. Untreated Dental Caries (Cavities) in Children Ages 2–19, United States. Available at: http://www.cdc.gov/Features/dsUntreatedCavitiesKids/.)

Oral cancer is the seventh most common cancer among men in the United States.[44] In the United States approximately 37,000 new cases of oral cancer are diagnosed annually and more than 8000 deaths are due to oral cancer.[45,46] In 2012 the number of new cases is expected to go up to 40,250 because of the increase in numbers of older adults. About 90% of these cases are squamous cell carcinomas, and the overall 5-year survival rate for oral cancer is approximately 50%.[47] The rates among women are lower when compared with men; however, recent trends show an increase in the incidence among women. Oral cancer occurs most commonly in adults aged 40 years and older. Oral diseases are expensive; each year in the United States approximately 500 million visits to the dental office are reported,[40] resulting in about $108 billion in national expenditures for dental services.

THE FUTURE BURDEN OF CHRONIC DISEASE PREVALENCE: PROJECTING TO 2050

Tables 3–14 show the population and prevalence estimates of the major chronic diseases projected to 2050. The population estimates are based on the US Bureau of Census trends, which have been demonstrated to be reliable.[48] According to the 2010 Census briefs, the older population grew at a faster rate between 2000 and 2010. Therefore it is unlikely that the projected population estimates are overestimates. The prevalence rates in the projected years are based on the currently observed prevalence rates. If disease rates decline, the projected prevalence in 2050 will be an overestimate. However, if disease rates increase these projected prevalences in 2050 will be an underestimate. The trends documented in the previous sections of this article show that prevalence rates have been increasing over the most recent 20 years for the chronic diseases analyzed here. If this trend continues, the projections calculated in this section will probably be underestimates. Moreover, with significant aging of the population the burden of chronic disease is more likely to be higher.

Methods

The population estimates for 2010 to 2050 are based on the US Bureau of Census population trends.[48] For the selected chronic diseases the most recent prevalence rates were obtained from data that are based on national health surveys and/or registries. The projected prevalence rates for each chronic disease were calculated by

Table 3
Projections for diagnosis of heart disease (all types) for the total population, by gender and selected age groups, using current prevalence rates and US Census Bureau population projections

Heart Disease (All Types)

	2010		2020		2040		2050	
	Population (Millions)	Prevalence (%)	Population (Millions)	No. with Disease (Millions)	Population (Millions)	No. with Disease (Millions)	Population (Millions)	No. with Disease (Millions)
Total	308.7	11.5	335.8	38.6	392.0	45.1	419.9	48.3
Male	151.8	13.2	165.1	21.7	192.4	25.4	206.6	27.3
Female	157.0	10.2	170.7	17.4	200.0	20.4	213.5	21.8
Age groups (years)								
20–44	103.7	4.4	89.0	3.9	101.6	4.5	109.3	4.8
45–64	81.5	13.1	83.7	10.9	88.6	11.6	93.1	12.2
65+	40.3	31.3	54.6	17.1	80.1	25.1	86.7	27.1

Table 4

Projections for diagnosis of coronary heart disease for the total population, by gender and selected age groups using current prevalence rates and US Census Bureau population projections

	Coronary Heart Disease								
	2010			2020		2040		2050	
	Population (Millions)	Prevalence (%)	No. with Disease (Millions)	Population (Millions)	No. with Disease (Millions)	Population (Millions)	No. with Disease (Millions)	Population (Millions)	No. with Disease (Millions)
Total	308.7	6.3	19.5	335.8	21.2	392.0	24.7	419.9	26.5
Male	151.8	8.4	12.7	165.1	14.0	192.4	16.2	206.6	17.3
Female	157.0	4.6	7.2	170.7	7.9	200.0	9.2	213.5	9.8
Age groups (years)									
20–44	103.7	1.1	1.1	89.0	1.0	101.6	1.1	109.3	1.2
45–64	81.5	7.2	5.9	83.7	6.0	88.6	6.4	93.1	6.7
65+	40.3	21.1	8.5	54.6	11.5	80.1	16.9	86.7	18.3

Table 5
Projections for diagnosis of stroke for the total population, by gender and selected age groups using current prevalence rates and US Census Bureau population projections

| | Stroke | | | | | | | | |
| | 2010 | | 2020 | | 2040 | | 2050 | | |
	Population (Millions)	Prevalence (%)	Population (Millions)	No. with Disease (Millions)	Population (Millions)	No. with Disease (Millions)	Population (Millions)	No. with Disease (Millions)
Total	308.7	2.6	335.8	8.7	392.0	10.2	419.9	10.9
Male	151.8	2.6	165.1	4.3	192.4	5.0	206.6	5.4
Female	157.0	2.6	170.7	4.4	200.0	5.2	213.5	5.5
Age groups (years)								
20–44	103.7	0.6	89.0	0.5	101.6	0.6	109.3	0.7
45–64	81.5	2.5	83.7	2.1	88.6	2.2	93.1	2.3
65+	40.3	9.2	54.6	5.0	80.1	7.4	86.7	8.0

Table 6
Projections for diagnosis of diabetes for the total population, by gender and selected age groups using current prevalence rates and US Census Bureau population projections

| | Diabetes | | | | | | | | | | | |
| | 2009 | | | 2010 | | 2020 | | 2040 | | 2050 | | |
	Population (Millions)	Prevalence (%)	No. with Diabetes (Millions)	Population (Millions)	No. with Diabetes (Millions)	Population (Millions)	No. with Diabetes (Millions)	Population (Millions)	No. with Diabetes (Millions)	Population (Millions)	No. with Diabetes (Millions)
Total	307.0	6.2	19.0	308.7	19.1	335.8	20.8	392.0	24.3	419.9	26.0
Male	151.5	6.6	10.0	151.8	10.0	165.1	11.0	192.4	12.7	206.6	13.6
Female	155.6	5.9	9.2	157.0	9.3	170.7	10.1	200.0	11.8	213.5	12.6
Age groups (years)											
0–44	188.1	1.7	3.2	103.7	3.3	89.0	3.4	101.6	3.8	109.3	4.1
45–64	79.4	12.2	9.7	81.5	9.9	83.7	10.2	88.6	10.8	93.1	11.4
65+	39.6	18.9	7.5	40.3	7.6	54.6	10.3	80.1	15.1	86.7	16.4

Table 7
Projections for diagnosis of lifetime asthma for the total population, by gender and selected age groups using current prevalence rates and US. Census Bureau population projections

Asthma (Lifetime)

	2009			2010		2020		2040		2050	
	Population (Millions)	Prevalence (%)	No. with Disease (Millions)	Population (Millions)	No. with Disease (Millions)	Population (Millions)	No. with Disease (Millions)	Population (Millions)	No. with Disease (Millions)	Population (Millions)	No. with Disease (Millions)
Overall	307.0	13.3	40.8	308.7	41.1	335.8	44.7	392.0	52.1	419.9	55.8
Male	151.5	12.6	19.1	151.8	19.1	165.1	20.8	192.4	24.2	206.6	26.0
Female	155.6	13.9	21.6	157.0	21.8	170.7	23.7	200.0	27.7	213.5	30.0
Age groups (years)											
<20	188.1	13.6	5.5	103.7	11.3	89.0	12.1	101.6	13.8	109.3	14.8
20–64	79.4	14.7	13.5	81.5	27.3	83.7	28.3	88.6	30.9	93.1	32.9
65+	39.6	11.3	4.5	40.3	4.6	54.6	6.2	80.1	9.1	86.7	10.0

Table 8

Projections for diagnosis of current asthma for the total population, by gender and selected age groups using current prevalence rates and US Census Bureau population projections

| | 2009 | | | 2010 | | 2020 | | 2040 | | 2050 | |
	Population (Millions)	Prevalence (%)	No. with Disease (Millions)	Population (Millions)	No. with Disease (Millions)	Population (Millions)	No. with Disease (Millions)	Population (Millions)	No. with Disease (Millions)	Population (Millions)	No. with Disease (Millions)
							Asthma (Current)				
Overall	307.0	8.2	25.2	308.7	25.3	335.8	27.5	392.0	32.1	419.9	34.4
Male	151.5	7.0	10.6	151.8	10.6	165.1	11.6	192.4	13.5	206.6	14.5
Female	155.6	9.3	14.5	157.0	14.6	170.7	15.9	200.0	18.6	213.5	19.8
Age groups (years)											
<20	188.1	8.6	3.5	103.7	7.2	89.0	7.6	101.6	8.7	109.3	9.4
20–64	79.4	7.7	7.1	81.5	14.3	83.7	14.8	88.6	16.2	93.1	17.3
65+	39.6	7.7	3.1	40.3	3.1	54.6	4.2	80.1	6.2	86.7	6.7

Table 9
Projections of overweight and obesity for the total population using current prevalence rates from BRFSS and US Census Bureau population projections

BRFSS data	2009			2010		2020		2040		2050	
	Population (Millions)	Prevalence (%)	No. with Disease (Millions)	Population (Millions)	No. with Disease (Millions)	Population (Millions)	No. with Disease (Millions)	Population (Millions)	No. with Disease (Millions)	Population (Millions)	No. with Disease (Millions)
Overweight: BMI 25–29.9											
Overall	307.0	27.2	83.5	308.7	84.0	335.8	91.3	391.9	106.6	419.9	114.2
Obese: BMI 30+											
Overall	307.0	36.2	111.1	308.7	111.8	335.8	121.6	391.9	141.9	419.9	152.0

Table 10
Projections of overweight and obesity combined for the total population, by gender and <20 years of age using current prevalence rates from NHANES and US Census Bureau population projections

NHANES 2007–2008	2009			2010		2020		2040		2050	
	Population (Millions)	Prevalence (%)	No. with Disease (Millions)	Population (Millions)	No. with Disease (Millions)	Population (Millions)	No. with Disease (Millions)	Population (Millions)	No. with Disease (Millions)	Population (Millions)	No. with Disease (Millions)
Overweight and Obesity Combined: BMI 25+											
Total	223.6	68.0	152.0	225.5	153.3	246.9	167.9	290.3	197.4	310.7	211.3
(age 20 and above)											
Male (20+)	108.7	72.3	78.6	109.2	78.9	119.7	86.5	140.5	101.6	150.7	109.0
Female (20+)	114.8	64.1	73.6	116.3	74.5	127.2	81.5	149.8	96.1	160.0	102.6
<20 y	40.7	17.8	7.2	83.3	14.8	88.9	15.8	101.6	18.1	109.1	19.4

Table 11

Projections for untreated dental caries for the total population, by selected age groups and gender using 2005–2008 prevalence rates from NHANES and US Census Bureau population projections

Percent of Untreated Dental Caries

	NHANES 2005–2008 Prevalence (%)	2010 Population (Millions)	2010 No. with Disease (Millions)	2020 Population (Millions)	2020 No. with Disease (Millions)	2040 Population (Millions)	2040 No. with Disease (Millions)	2050 Population (Millions)	2050 No. with Disease (Millions)
6–19 y	16.1	57.6	9.3	61.4	9.9	70.2	11.3	75.5	12.2
Male	17	29.5	5.0	31.4	5.3	35.9	6.1	38.6	6.6
Female	15.3	28.1	4.3	30.0	4.6	34.3	5.2	36.9	5.6
20–64 y	23.2	185.5	43.0	192.3	44.6	210.3	48.8	224.0	52.0
Male	26.6	92.2	24.5	95.9	25.5	105.4	28.0	112.4	29.9
Female	19.9	93.2	18.5	96.4	19.2	104.9	20.9	111.6	22.2
65–74 y	18.3	21.3	3.9	31.8	5.8	35.5	6.5	37.9	6.9
Male	22.9	9.8	2.2	14.8	3.4	16.8	3.8	18.2	4.2
Female	14.6	11.5	1.7	17.0	2.5	18.7	2.7	19.8	2.9
75+ y	17.7	19.0	3.4	22.9	4.1	44.6	7.9	48.8	8.6
Male	22.1	7.2	1.6	9.0	2.0	18.3	4.0	20.1	4.4
Female	14.3	11.8	1.7	13.9	2.0	26.3	3.8	28.6	4.1

Table 12

Projections for diagnosis of periodontal disease for the total population, by selected age groups and gender using 1999-2004 NHANES prevalence rates and US Census Bureau population projections

Prevalence of Periodontal Disease

NHANES 1999–2004	Periodontal Disease	2010		2020		2040		2050	
	Prevalence (%)	Population (Millions)	No. with Disease (Millions)	Population (Millions)	No. with Disease (Millions)	Population (Millions)	No. with Disease (Millions)	Population (Millions)	No. with Disease (Millions)
Age (years)									
20–34	3.84	63.3	2.4	65.8	2.5	74.7	2.9	79.1	3.0
35–49	10.41	63.8	6.6	63.0	6.6	70.8	7.4	76.3	7.9
50–64	11.88	58.4	6.9	63.4	7.5	64.9	7.7	68.6	8.2
65–74	10.20	21.3	2.2	31.8	3.2	35.5	3.6	37.9	3.9
75+	11.03	19.0	2.1	22.9	2.5	44.6	4.9	48.8	5.4
20–64									
Male	10.65	92.2	9.8	95.9	10.2	105.4	11.2	112.4	12.0
Female	6.40	93.2	6.0	96.4	6.2	104.9	6.7	111.6	7.1
65+									
Male	12.97	17.0	2.2	23.7	3.1	35.1	4.5	38.3	5.0
Female	8.56	23.2	2.0	30.9	2.6	45.0	3.9	48.4	4.1

Table 13
Projections for diagnosis of moderate or severe periodontal disease for the total population, by selected age groups and gender using 1999-2004 NHANES prevalence rates and US Census Bureau population projections

| | NHANES 1999–2004 Moderate or Severe Periodontal Disease | Prevalence of Moderate or Severe Periodontal Disease | | | | | | | |
| | | 2010 | | 2020 | | 2040 | | 2050 | |
Age (years)	Prevalence (%)	Population (Millions)	No. with Disease (Millions)	Population (Millions)	No. with Disease (Millions)	Population (Millions)	No. with Disease (Millions)	Population (Millions)	No. with Disease (Millions)
20–34	n/a	63.3		65.8		74.7		79.1	
35–49	5.0	63.8	3.2	63.0	3.2	70.8	3.5	76.3	3.8
50–64	10.7	58.4	6.3	63.4	6.8	64.9	7.0	68.6	7.4
65–74	14.3	21.3	3.0	31.8	4.5	35.5	5.1	37.9	5.4
75+	20.8	19.0	3.9	22.9	4.7	44.6	9.3	48.8	10.1
20–64									
Male	6.7	92.2	6.2	95.9	6.5	105.4	7.1	112.4	7.6
Female	3.5	93.2	3.2	96.4	3.3	104.9	3.6	111.6	3.9
65+									
Male	20.6	17.0	3.5	23.7	4.9	35.1	7.2	38.3	7.9
Female	14.4	23.2	3.3	30.9	4.4	45.0	6.5	48.4	7.0

Table 14
Projections for diagnosis of oral cancer for the total population, by gender and selected age groups using 2008 SEER 11* prevalence rates and US Census Bureau population projections

2008 SEER 11 Population	Prevalence (%)	Oral Cancer							
		2010		2020		2040		2050	
		Population (Millions)	No. with Disease (Millions)	Population (Millions)	No. with Disease (Millions)	Population Millions	No. with Disease (Millions)	Population (Millions)	No. with Disease (Millions)
Total	0.06	308.7	0.18	335.8	0.19	392.0	0.22	420.0	0.24
Gender									
Male	0.08	151.8	0.12	165.1	0.13	192.4	0.16	206.5	0.17
Female	0.04	157.0	0.06	170.7	0.06	200.0	0.07	213.4	0.08
Age groups (years)									
30–39	0.01	40.4	0.006	44.8	0.007	48.8	0.007	52.8	0.008
40–49	0.04	43.6	0.02	40.9	0.02	46.7	0.02	50.0	0.02
50–59	0.12	41.7	0.05	42.6	0.05	45.1	0.05	46.3	0.05
60–69	0.19	28.9	0.06	38.5	0.07	38.0	0.07	42.8	0.08
70–79	0.22	16.3	0.04	23.6	0.05	33.4	0.07	32.6	0.07
80+	0.20	11.8	0.02	13.4	0.03	28.4	0.06	33.7	0.07

multiplying the US Census Bureau population estimates by current prevalence rates for that chronic illness. Projection estimates were calculated according to gender and selected age groups. The methods used here are similar to those used in similar projection studies.[49–51] Projections are presented here for coronary heart disease, stroke, diabetes, asthma, overweight, and oral diseases.

Heart Disease

At present, 11.5%, or 33.5 million people, have some type of cardiovascular disease (see **Table 3**). As the United States population increases to more than 400 million in 2050, there will be 48.3 million people (27.2 million males and 21.1 million females) with some type of cardiovascular disease. The over-65 age group has the highest rate at 31.3%, which means that there will be 27.1 million seniors older than 65 with cardiovascular disease.

Coronary heart disease (CHD) is the most common form of cardiovascular disease, with 6.3% of the entire population and 21.2% of the senior population older than 65 years having been diagnosed with this chronic condition (see **Table 4**). The number of older adults (65+) with CHD grows from 11.5 million in 2020 to 18.3 million in 2050.

Stroke

Table 5 shows that the prevalence of stroke will increase from 8 million people in 2010 to 11 million people in 2050. Males and females are about equal in their experience with stroke. However, stroke prevalence increases dramatically with age, to 9.2% of the over-65 age group. This trend will significantly affect the health care burden as stroke patients, particularly the elderly, use significant amounts of medical system resources.

Diabetes

In 2009 a total of 19 million persons were diagnosed with diabetes among the United States population of 307 million (see **Table 6**). By the year 2050 the prevalence of diabetes is projected to be 26 million. In 2050 males are predicted to have a higher prevalence (13.6 million) compared with females (12.6 million). This trend is probably due to the predicted demographic increase in the male population among those 65 years and older as the population ages. The highest diabetes prevalence is expected among those 65 years and older. Earlier studies on projection of diabetes prevalence have reported a projected estimate of more than 29 million in 2050.[49]

Asthma

Tables 7 and **8** show projected estimates for lifetime and current asthma prevalence rates, respectively. Lifetime asthma sufferers will increase from 40.8 million in 2009 to 55.8 million in 2050. Females are projected to have higher prevalence (29 million) in comparison with males (26 million). Current asthma diagnosis will increase from 25 million in 2009 to 34 million in 2050. Asthma is clearly trending toward becoming a significant challenge for the United States health care system.

Overweight and Obesity

According to national survey data from the 2009 BRFSS, currently more than 83 million people are overweight (BMI 25–29.9). In 2050 this is projected to increase to an astounding 114 million (see **Table 9**). Obesity prevalence is predicted to be higher with a projected estimate of 151 million in 2050, which is 36% higher than the current estimate of 111 million (see **Table 10**). Based on prevalence data from NHANES, the combined prevalence of overweight and obesity (BMI 25 and above) is currently more than 152 million (see **Table 10**), with a projected to increase to more than 211 million in 2050. Prevalence is projected to be almost equal among males (109 million) and females (103 million).

Oral Disease

The prevalence of untreated dental caries was reported to be 16.1% in the NHANES data from 2005 to 2008 (see **Table 11**). The highest prevalence was among males and adults aged 20 to 64 years. Based on these rates, the projected increase in prevalence of untreated dental caries in 2050 is expected to increase by 33%.

Prevalence rates for periodontal disease reported in NHANES from 1999 to 2004 show higher prevalence among males aged 65 years and older (see **Table 12**). In 2010, when analyzing by age the prevalence is highest among those aged 35 to 64 years. When evaluating by age and gender, in 2010 among males aged 20 to 64 years 9.8 million are estimated to have periodontal disease in comparison with 6 million among females aged 20 to 64 years. In 2050 this difference in estimates between males and females is expected to increase further, with projected estimates of 12 million among males and 7 million among females. For moderate or severe periodontal disease the prevalence estimates in 2050 are projected to be highest among those aged 75 years and older (see **Table 13**). Among those aged 20 to 64 years, 7.6 million males are projected to have moderate or severe periodontal disease in comparison with 3.9 million females. As age increases, the prevalence (ie, among those 65 years and older) estimates become more similar among males and females. Oral cancer prevalence projections were calculated based on SEER 11 prevalence rates. Overall the projected prevalence for oral cancer in 2050 is expected to be 33% higher than the estimated current prevalence (**Table 14**) particularly among males (42% increase).

SUMMARY OF CHRONIC DISEASE PROJECTIONS

At present, 11.5%, or 33.5 million people, have some type of cardiovascular disease (see **Table 5**). However, as the population increases to more than 400 million in 2050, there will be 48.3 million people (27.2 million males and 21.1 million females) with some type of cardiovascular disease. Most of these will comprise 27.1 million seniors older than 65 years. CHD is the most common form of cardiovascular disease, and among those aged 65 years and older 21.2% have been diagnosed with this chronic condition (see **Table 6**). Stroke is the third leading cause of death in the United States, and currently 8 million adults have been diagnosed with stroke. The prevalence of stroke increases dramatically with age, to 9.2% of the over-65 age group, which will significantly affect the health care burden resulting from overuse of medical system resources.

In 2050 males are predicted to have a higher prevalence (13.6 million) of diabetes compared with females (12.6 million). This trend is probably due to the predicted increase in the male population among those 65 years and older as the population ages. Asthma rates are also projected to increase. The number of persons with lifetime asthma will increase, from 40.8 million in 2009 to 55.8 million in 2050. Females are projected to have higher prevalence (29 million) than males (26 million). Obesity increases the risk for most chronic diseases. Obesity prevalence is predicted to be high, with a projected estimate of 151 million in 2050, which is 36% higher than the current estimate of 111 million (see **Table 10**). Based on prevalence data from NHANES, the combined prevalence of overweight and obesity (BMI 25 and above) is currently more than 152 million (see **Table 10**), which is projected to increase to more than

Table 15
Number of people with chronic disease by year (in millions)

Chronic Disease	Currently (2010)	The Future (2050)
Heart disease (all types)	35.5	48.3
CHD	19.5	26.5
Stroke	8.0	10.9
Diabetes	19	26
Asthma, lifetime	40.8	55.8
Asthma, current	25.2	34.4
Obesity (BMI 30+)	111.1	152.0
Obesity and overweight combined (BMI 25+)	152.0	211.3
Dental caries	Ages 20–64 y: 9.3	Ages 20–64 y: 12.2
Periodontal disease	Males vs females: 9.8 vs 6	Males vs females: 12 vs 7

211 million in 2050. The projected increase in prevalence of untreated dental caries in 2050 is expected to be 12.2 million, in comparison with an estimate of 9.3 million in 2010. The current difference in prevalence for moderate periodontal disease among males versus females is predicted to further widen by 2050, with males predicted to have a higher prevalence. Older males are predicted to have much higher prevalence of severe periodontal disease as well (**Table 15**).

Overall, the data presented here clearly show that obesity by itself and obesity combined with overweight are going to be the greatest burden on public health and medical resources as they significantly increase the risks of diabetes, heart disease, high blood pressure, arthritis, stroke, and some cancers (**Fig. 19**). The projected estimates that for the major chronic diseases such as heart disease, diabetes, and stroke are based on current prevalence rates. However, one can expect an even higher prevalence of these diseases by 2050 as a result of the high prevalence of obesity.

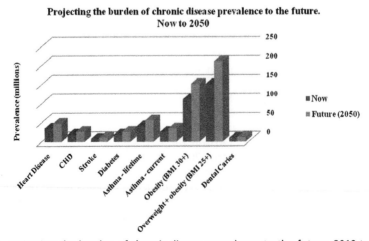

Fig. 19. Projecting the burden of chronic disease prevalence to the future, 2010 to 2050.

SUMMARY

1. Chronic diseases are the major causes of death among adults in the United States.
2. Prevalence of chronic disease increases with age.
3. The United States population is aging rapidly.
4. The prevalence of chronic diseases will increase as the population grows and ages.
5. The management of chronic illnesses will become an increasing burden for primary care providers.
6. In the future dentists will be expected to monitor chronic disease and control the risk factors (ie, provide primary care) for levels of chronic disease in their own dental patients.[50,51]

REFERENCES

1. National Center for Health Statistics Health, United States, 2008. Hyattsville (MD): Chart book; 2009. Available at: http://www.cdc.gov/nchs/hus.htm. Accessed November 7, 2011.
2. Werner C. 2011. The Older Population: 2010. U.S. Census Bureau; 2012. Available at: http://www.census.gov/prod/cen2010/briefs/c2010br-09.pdf.
3. NCHS. National Center for Health Statistics. Health, United States, 2007. With chart book on trends in the health of Americans. Hyattsville (MD): National Center for Health Statistics; 2007. Available at: http://wwwcdcgov/nchs/data/hus/hus07pdf. Accessed October 25, 2011.
4. Day J. National population projections. US Census Bureau; 2001. Available at: http://wwwcensusgov/population/www/pop-profile/natprojhtml. Accessed November 9, 2011.
5. Kung H, Hoyert D, Xu J, et al. Deaths: final data for 2005. Natl Vital Stat Rep 2008; 56(10). Available at: http://wwwcdcgov/nchs/data/nvsr/nvsr56/nvsr56_10pdf. Accessed November 3, 2011.
6. Anderson G. Chronic conditions: making the case for ongoing care. Baltimore (MD): John Hopkins University; 2004.
7. National health expenditures aggregate, per capita amounts, percent distribution, and average annual percent growth, by source of funds: selected calendar years 1960-2007 [internet]. Baltimore (MD): Centers for Medicare and Medicaid Services; 2008. Available at: http://www.cms.hhs.gov/NationalHealthExpend Data/downloads/tables.pdf. Accessed February 17, 2012.
8. CDC. Chronic diseases and health promotion. Centers for Disease Control and Prevention; 2011. Available at: http://www.cdc.gov/chronicdisease/overview/index.htm. Accessed October 25, 2011.
9. Kochanek K, Xu J, Murphy S. Deaths: preliminary data for 2009; National vital statistics reports, vol. 59. Hyattsville (MD): National Center for Health Statistics; 2011.
10. Wu S, Green A. Projection of chronic illness prevalence and cost inflation. Santa Monica (CA): RAND Health; 2000.
11. DeVol R, Bedroussian A. An unhealthy America: the economic burden of chronic disease [executive summary and research findings]. 2007. Available at: www.milkeninstitute.org. Accessed November 14, 2011.
12. Anderson G, Horvath J. The growing burden of chronic disease in America. Public Health Rep 2004;119:263–70.
13. Van Cleave J, Gortmaker S, Perrin J. Dynamics of obesity and chronic health conditions among children and youth. JAMA 2010;303:623–30.
14. Lloyd-Jones D, Adams R, Brown T. Heart disease and stroke statistics—2010 update. A report from the American Heart Association Statistics Committee and

Stroke Statistics Subcommittee external web site icon. Circulation 2010;121: e1–170.

15. Roger V, Go A, Lloyd-Jones D, et al. Heart disease and stroke statistics-2011 update. A report from the American Heart Association. Circulation 2011;123: e18–209.

16. Heron M, Hoyert D, Murphy S, et al. Deaths: final data for 2006 Adobe PDF file [PDF-2.3M]. National Vital Statistics Reports, vol. 57. Hyattsville (MD): National Center for Health Statistics; 2009.

17. CDC. Racial/ethnic and socioeconomic disparities in multiple risk factors for heart disease and stroke-United States, 2003. MMWR Morb Mortal Wkly Rep 2005;54: 113–7. Available at: http://wwwcdcgov/mmwr/preview/mmwrhtml/mm5405a1htm. Accessed November 10, 2011.

18. CDC. Prevalence of coronary heart disease—United States, 2006-2010. MMWR Morb Mortal Wkly Rep 2011;60:1377–81.

19. Howlader N, Noone A, Krapcho M, et al. SEER cancer statistics review, 1975-2008. Bethesda (MD): National Cancer Institute; 2011. Available at: http://seer.cancer.gov/csr/1975_2008/. Accessed March 5, 2012.

20. Cancer facts and figures, 2011. American Cancer Society 2011. Available at: http://wwwcancerorg/acs/groups/content/@epidemiologysurveilance/documents/document/acspc-029771pdf. Accessed November 10, 2011.

21. Pleis JR, Ward BW, Lucas JW. Summary health statistics for U.S. adults: National Health Interview Survey, 2009. Vital Health Stat 2010;249:1–207.

22. American Cancer Society. Cancer facts & figures 2008. Atlanta (GA): American Cancer Society; 2008. Available at: http://www.cancer.org/docroot/stt/content/stt_1x_cancer_facts_and_figures_2008.asp. Accessed November 10, 2011.

23. The health consequences of smoking: a report of the surgeon general. Atlanta (GA): U.S. Department of Health and Human Services, Centers for Disease Control and Prevention; 2004. Available at: http://www.cdc.gov/tobacco/data_statistics/sgr/sgr_2004/index.htm. Accessed November 10, 2011.

24. Rosamond W, Flegal K, Friday G. Heart disease and stroke statistics—2007 update: a report from the American Heart Association Statistics Committee and Stroke Statistics Subcommittee. Circulation 2007;115:e69–171.

25. BRFSS. Behavioral Risk Factor Surveillance System. 2011. Available at: http://appsnccdcdcgov/brfss/pageasp?yr=2010&state=US&cat=DB#DB. Accessed October 24, 2011.

26. American Diabetes Association. Standards of medical care in diabetes. Diabetes Care 2009;32:S13–61.

27. CDC. National diabetes fact sheet: national estimates and general information on diabetes and prediabetes in the United States, 2011. Atlanta (GA): U.S. Department of Health and Human Services, Centers for Disease Control and Prevention; 2011.

28. CDC. National diabetes fact sheet 2007. Atlanta (GA): U.S. Department of Health and Human Services; 2008. Available at: http://www.cdc.gov/Diabetes/pubs/factsheet07.htm. Accessed November 9, 2011.

29. Fox C, Pencina M, Meigs J, et al. Trends in the incidence of type 2 diabetes mellitus from the 1970s to the 1990s: the Framingham Heart Study. Circulation 2006; 113:2914–8.

30. Vital signs: asthma prevalence, disease characteristics, and self-management education—United States, 2001-2009. MMWR Morb Mortal Wkly Rep 2011;60: 547–52.

31. WHO. Obesity: preventing and managing the global epidemic. Report of a World Health Organization (WHO) Consultation. Geneva, 2000. WHO Technical Report Series, 2000; 894.

32. Flegal KM, Carroll MD, Ogden CL, et al. Prevalence and trends in obesity among US adults, 1999-2008. JAMA 2010;303:235–41.

33. CDC. Overweight and obesity: U.S. Obesity trends. Centers for Disease Control and Prevention (CDC); 2011. Available at: http://wwwcdcgov/obesity/data/trendshtml. Accessed December 4, 2011.

34. NIH. NHLBI Obesity Education Initiative. Clinical guidelines on the identification, evaluation, and treatment of overweight and obesity in adults. National Institutes of Health 1998;98–4083. Available at: http://www.nhlbi.nih.gov/guidelines/obesity/ob_gdlns.pdfExternal. Accessed December 4, 2011.

35. Finkelstein E, Trogdon J, Cohen J, et al. Annual medical spending attributable to obesity: payer- and service-specific estimates. Health Aff 2009;28:w822–31.

36. Wolf A. What is the economic case for treating obesity? Obes Res 1998;6:2S–7S.

37. Wolf A, Colditz G. Current estimates of the economic cost of obesity in the United States. Obes Res 1998;6:97–106.

38. Dye B, Tan S, Smith V, et al. Trends in oral health status: United States, 1988-1994 and 1999-2004. Vital and Health Statistics; 2007. Available at: http://www.cdc.gov/nchs/data/series/sr_11/sr11_248.pdf. 11. Accessed November 10, 2011.

39. The burden of oral disease: tool for creating state documents. Atlanta (GA): U.S. Department of Health and Human Services; 2005. Available at: http://wwwcdcgov/oralhealth/library/burdenbook/. Accessed November 10, 2011.

40. Oral health: preventing cavities, gum disease, tooth loss, and oral cancers at a glance. National Center for Chronic Disease Prevention and Health Promotion, Division of Oral Health, Centers for Disease Control and Prevention, Atlanta, Georgia; 2011. Available at: http://www.cdc.gov/chronicdisease/resources/publications/aag/pdf/2011/Oral-Health-AAG-PDF-508.pdf.

41. CDC Centers for Disease Control and Prevention. The burden of oral disease: tool for creating state documents. Atlanta (GA): U.S. Department of Health and Human Services; 2005. Available at: http://www.cdc.gov/oralhealth/library/burdenbook/. 2005. Accessed November 10, 2011.

42. Borrell L, Burt B, Taylor G. Prevalence and trends in periodontitis in the USA: from NHANES III to the NHANES, 1988 to 2000. J Dent Res 2005;84:924–30.

43. Joshipura K, Ritchie C, Douglass C. Strength of evidence linking oral conditions and systemic diseases. Journal - Compendium of Continuing Education in Dentistry 2000;(Suppl 30):12–23.

44. Ries LAG, Eisner MP, Kosary CL. SEER Cancer Statistics Review, 1975-2001. Bethesda, MD: National Cancer Institute; 2004. Available at: http://seer.cancer.gov/csr/1975_2001.

45. Oral Cancer. American Cancer Society 2007. Rev. 02/12. Page accessed March 2012. Available at: http://www.cancer.org/acs/groups/content/@nho/documents/document/oralcancerpdf.pdf. Accessed November 7, 2011.

46. Kujan OG, Oliver R, Thakker N, et al. Screening programmes for the early detection and prevention of oral cancer. Cochrane Database Syst Rev 2006;(3):CD004150.

47. SEER. Cancer statistics, 2011. Available at: http://seercancergov/statfacts/html/oralcavhtml. Accessed December 4, 2011.

48. Howden LM, Meyer JA. Age and Sex Composition: 2010. United States Census Bureau. Accessed at: http://www.census.gov/prod/cen2010/briefs/c2010br-03.pdf. Accessed December 3, 2011.

49. Boyle J, Geiss L, Honeycutt A, et al. Projection of diabetes burden through 2050: impact of changing demography and disease prevalence in the U.S. Diabetes Care 2001;24:1936–40.

50. Greenberg B, Glick M, Frantsve-Hawley J, et al. Dentists' attitudes toward chair-side screening for medical conditions. J Am Dent Assoc 2010;141(1):52–62. Available at: Ipswich (MA): Dentistry & Oral Sciences Source. Available at: http://vufind.carli.illinois.edu/vf-uiu/Record/uiu_6688087/Description. Accessed June 18, 2012.

51. Lalla E, Kaplan S, Chang SM, et al. Periodontal infection profiles in type 1 diabetes. J Clin Periodontol 2006;33:855–62.

The Assessment and Importance of Hypertension in the Dental Setting

Jonathan Hogan, MD, Jai Radhakrishnan, MD, MS, MRCP, FASN*

KEYWORDS

- Hypertension • Blood pressure • Antihypertensive drugs • Cardiovascular effects

KEY POINTS

- Many patients with hypertension have uncontrolled disease. The dental visit presents a unique opportunity to screen patients for undiagnosed and undertreated hypertension, which may lead to improved monitoring and treatment.
- Although there are no clinical studies, it is generally recommended that nonemergent procedures be avoided in patients with a blood pressure of greater than 180/110 mm Hg.
- Because of the high prevalence of disease and medication use for hypertension, dentists should be aware of the oral side effects of antihypertensive medications as well as the cardiovascular effects of medications commonly used during dental visits.

HYPERTENSION: DEFINITION, IMPORTANCE, AND BENEFITS OF TREATMENT

The most commonly referenced guideline pertaining to blood pressure in adults in the United Sates is the Seventh Report of the Joint National Committee on the Prevention, Detection, Evaluation, and Treatment of High Blood Pressure (JNC 7),[1] which was published in 2003. JNC 7 defines hypertension as a systolic blood pressure (SBP) greater than 140 mm Hg or a diastolic blood pressure (DBP) greater than 90 mm Hg. These definitions are derived from studies showing increased adverse cardiovascular outcomes in patients with blood pressure above these levels. A meta-analysis demonstrated that for each 20 mm Hg increase of SBP above 115 mm Hg and 10 mm Hg of DBP 75 mm Hg in patients 40 to 70 years of age, the risk of death from cardiovascular events (stroke, myocardial infarction) doubles (**Fig. 1**).[2] JNC 7 also introduced the category of Prehypertension, which is defined as an SBP of 120 to 139 mm Hg and DBP of 80 to 89 mm Hg (**Table 1**). These individuals are at increased risk of developing hypertension.

Division of Nephrology, Department of Medicine, Columbia University College of Physician and Surgeons, 622 West 168th Street, PH 4-124, New York, NY 10032, USA
* Corresponding author.
E-mail address: jr55@columbia.edu

Dent Clin N Am 56 (2012) 731–745
http://dx.doi.org/10.1016/j.cden.2012.07.003
0011-8532/12/$ – see front matter © 2012 Elsevier Inc. All rights reserved.

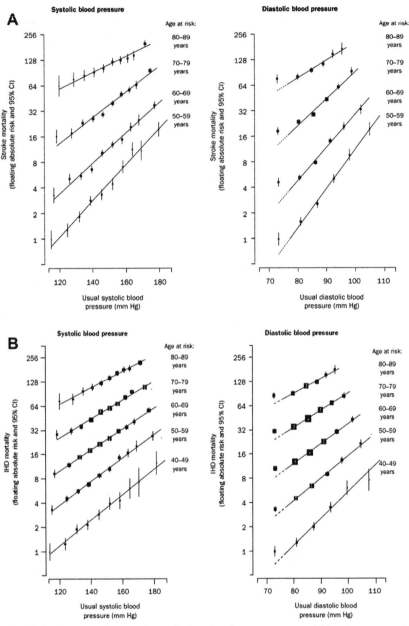

Fig. 1. (*A*) Stroke mortality rate in each decade of age versus usual blood pressure at the start of that decade. (*B*) Ischemic heart disease (IHD) mortality rate in each decade of age versus blood pressure at the start of that decade. CI, confidence interval. (*From* Lewington S, Clarke R, Qizilbash N, et al. Age-specific relevance of usual blood pressure to vascular mortality: a meta-analysis of individual data for one million adults in 61 prospective studies. Lancet 2002;360(9349):1903–13; with permission.)

Table 1
JNC 7 classifications of blood pressure

Classification	SBP (mm Hg)	DBP (mm Hg)
Normal	<120	And <80
Prehypertension	120–139	Or 80–89
Stage I hypertension	140–159	Or 90–99
Stage II hypertension	≥160	Or ≥100

Abbreviations: DBP, diastolic blood pressure; SBP, systolic blood pressure.
Data from Chobanian AV, Bakris GL, Black HR, et al. The Seventh Report of the Joint National Committee on Prevention, Detection, Evaluation, and Treatment of High Blood Pressure: the JNC 7 report. JAMA 2003;289(19):2560–72.

Treating hypertensive patients with lifestyle modification and medications has been associated with reductions in adverse cardiovascular outcomes. One meta-analysis showed a reduction of stroke by 30% to 39%, major cardiovascular events by 20% to 28%, and heart failure by more than 50% with the use of medications such as angiotensin-converting enzyme inhibitors (ACEIs) and calcium-channel blockers.[3] Physicians aim to achieve a goal blood pressure that is dependent on the patient's age and additional medical problems, if present.

EPIDEMIOLOGY

As of the publication of the JNC 7 report, an estimated 50 million Americans had hypertension, making it the most commonly diagnosed medical condition in the United States.[1] JNC 7 estimated that 1 billion people worldwide have hypertension. Furthermore, 30% of patients with hypertension were unaware that they had the condition, 41% were not being treated for their disease, and only 34% of patients had reached a goal blood pressure of less than 140/90 mm Hg. Screening for hypertension during dental visits, therefore, is an opportunity to increase hypertensive patients' awareness of their disease, as well as to improve medical referral for initiation or modification of treatment.

MEASUREMENT OF BLOOD PRESSURE

The gold standard for measurement of blood pressure is via an intra-arterial catheter. However, this is an invasive and impractical method to measure blood pressure in outpatients. The most common methods used to evaluate blood pressure are office blood pressure measurement, home blood pressure measurement (whereby a patient measures his/her blood pressure at home with a blood pressure machine), and ambulatory blood pressure measurement (whereby a patient's blood pressure is measured at intervals over a 24-hour period to calculate averages in SBP and DBP). A dentist's role in measuring blood pressure will likely be limited to office blood pressure measurements.

JNC 7 includes a description of the method that health care professionals should use to obtain office blood pressure measurements. One must use a properly calibrated and validated blood pressure instrument. Patients should be seated in a chair (not an examination table) with their feet on the floor for 5 minutes in a quiet room. Their arm should be supported at the level of the heart and an appropriately sized blood pressure cuff (cuff bladder encircling at least 80% of the arm) must be used. Accurate measurement of blood pressure is important to avoid overdiagnosis and underdiagnosis, as well as overtreatment and undertreatment, of hypertension. Although the use of noninvasive blood pressure measurements does lead to discrepancies compared with intra-arterial catheter measurement,[4] most large trials that have studied hypertension-related outcomes have been performed with the noninvasive technique, and it is currently still widely relied on.

WHITE-COAT HYPERTENSION, THE WHITE-COAT EFFECT, AND MASKED HYPERTENSION

White-coat hypertension (WCH) refers to a persistently elevated office blood pressure in the presence of a normal blood pressure outside of the office.[5,6] WCH is different from the white-coat effect (WCE), which refers to a high office blood pressure but whereby hypertension may or may not be present outside the office setting. Masked hypertension refers to when a patient has a normal office blood pressure but has hypertension outside of the office (**Table 2**). WCH, the WCE, and masked hypertension can be diagnosed through various methods including home blood pressure monitoring and 24-hour ambulatory blood pressure monitoring. WCH and masked hypertension are important for clinicians to recognize. It is controversial as to whether WCH is associated with increased cardiovascular risk,[7] but patients with masked hypertension are at increased cardiovascular risk. The prevalence of WHC during physician visits is approximately 20%.[6] The prevalence of WCH in the setting of visits to the dentist's office has not been established.

PATHOPHYSIOLOGIC MECHANISMS AND TREATMENT STRATEGIES FOR HYPERTENSION

It is important to first recognize that a subset of patients with elevated blood pressure will have secondary hypertension: hypertension that has an identifiable medical cause which, if corrected, will result in the resolution of high blood pressure. These causes include primary hyperaldosteronism, Cushing disease, coarctation of the aorta, pheochromocytoma, and renovascular hypertension. Ninety-five percent of patients, however, will have no identifiable cause for their hypertension; this is called essential hypertension and is the focus of the remainder of this section.

Essential hypertension has been shown to have many pathophysiological causes (**Table 3**). Three important causes are salt/volume overload, activation of the renin-angiotensin-aldosterone system (RAAS), and activation of the sympathetic nervous system. It is important that this physiology is understood, because most current pharmacologic and nonpharmacologic treatment is based on targeting these mechanisms.[8]

Salt/Volume Overload

Salt (sodium chloride) overload/volume overload is one mechanism that commonly contributes to essential hypertension. High sodium intake has been associated with essential hypertension in a variety of scientific models and clinical studies, and

Table 2
White-coat hypertension (WCH) versus white-coat effect (WCE) versus masked hypertension

Diagnosis	Office Blood Pressure	Blood Pressure Outside Office	Associated with Adverse Outcomes?
WCH	Elevated	Normal	Controversial
WCE	Elevated	Normal or High	Controversial
Masked hypertension	Normal	Elevated	Yes

Table 3
Three mechanisms known to contribute to essential hypertension, and antihypertensive medication classes targeting these mechanisms

Mechanism	Medications Targeting this Mechanism (Examples)
Volume overload	Diuretics (hydrochlorothiazide, chlorthalidone, metolazone, furosemide, torsemide)
	Dihydropyridine CCBs (amlodipine, nifedipine)
Renin-angiotensin-aldosterone system	ACEIs (lisinopril, captopril)
	ARBs (losartan, valsartan)
	β-Blockers (metoprolol, carvedilol)
	Direct renin inhibitors (aliskerin)
	Aldosterone receptor blockers (spironolactone, eplerenone)
Sympathetic nervous system	Central α-blockers (clonidine)
	Peripheral α-blockers (tamsulosin, terazosin)
	β-Blockers (metoprolol, carvedilol)
	Nondihydropyridine CCBs (verapamil, diltiazem)
	Vasodilators (minoxidil, hydralazine, nitrates)

Abbreviations: ACEI, angiotensin-converting enzyme inhibitor; ARB, angiotensin II receptor blocker; CCB, calcium-channel blocker.
Data from Chobanian AV, Bakris GL, Black HR, et al. The Seventh Report of the Joint National Committee on Prevention, Detection, Evaluation, and Treatment of High Blood Pressure: the JNC 7 report. JAMA 2003;289(19):2560–72.

decreasing the sodium intake ameliorates this effect.[9,10] High sodium intake increases blood pressure by expanding intravascular volume, and may have direct neurohormonal effects on the cardiovascular system.[10] Such salt-sensitive patients benefit from the following interventions:

- A low sodium diet (less than 2.4 g of sodium per day) or the DASH diet (Dietary Approaches to Stop Hypertension),[11] which is low in sodium and higher in other elements such as potassium and calcium.
- Diuretics, which are medications that increase urinary sodium excretion by blocking reabsorption of sodium in the kidney. Commonly used medications include loop diuretics (such as furosemide, bumetanide, and torsemide), thiazide and thiazide-like diuretics (such as hydrochlorothiazide, chlorthalidone, and metolazone), and aldosterone-receptor blockers (such as spironolactone and eplerenone). These classes of diuretics differ in their sites of action within the nephron.
- Calcium-channel blockers, which include dihydropyridines (peripheral-acting medications such as nifedipine and amlodipine) and nondihydropyridines (central-acting medications such as verapamil and diltiazem), which are vasodilators and have negative effects on cardiac output, and also are effective in patients with sodium and volume overload.

Renin-Angiotensin-Aldosterone System

The RAAS hormonal axis also contributes to hypertension in many patients. Renin, a hormone synthesized and released by the kidney in response to intravascular volume depletion and hyperkalemia, promotes the conversion of angiotensinogen (produced by the liver) to angiotensin I. Angiotensin I is then converted to angiotensin II by the angiotensin-converting enzyme (ACE) in the lung. Angiotensin II increases blood pressure by increasing renal sodium reabsorption, producing vasoconstriction, and activating the sympathetic nervous system (see later discussion). Angiotensin II also increases the production and secretion of aldosterone from the adrenal cortex.

Aldosterone also increases renal sodium reabsorption. Thus, the RAAS system increases blood pressure through increasing renal sodium reabsorption (which leads to intravascular volume expansion) and vasoconstriction (**Fig. 2**).

The RAAS is activated in many patients with essential hypertension and other associated conditions such as obesity and sleep apnea. In addition to treating these underlying diseases, medications are used to block various components of the RAAS pathway.

- β-Blockers such as propranolol, carvedilol, and metoprolol decrease renal renin release.
- The direct renin inhibitor aliskiren binds to renin and thus prevents the conversion of angiotensinogen to angiotensin I.
- ACEIs block ACE and therefore prevent the conversion of angiotensin I to angiotensin II.
- Angiotensin II receptor blockers (ARBs) prevent angiotensin II from binding to its receptor, decreasing vasoconstriction and renal sodium reabsorption.
- Aldosterone-receptor blockers (such as spironolactone and eplerenone) and other medications such as amiloride decrease the effects of aldosterone-mediated renal sodium reabsorption.

Sympathetic Nervous System

Activation of the sympathetic nervous system (SNS) also contributes to the development, maintenance, and progression of hypertension. There are many, incompletely understood mechanisms by which SNS activation leads to hypertension. SNS activation is present in many disease states such as obesity, obstructive sleep apnea, and alcoholism, and therapies have been developed to target the central, peripheral, and renal SNS to improve the control of blood pressure.

Therapies to improve blood pressure in these patients include:

- Treatment of underlying contributing conditions through weight loss, treatment of sleep apnea, and avoidance of alcohol, respectively
- Medications that mitigate the actions of an activated SNS such as peripheral α1-receptor blockers (such as terazosin and tamsulosin), the central α2-agonist clonidine, and β-blockers[1,8]
- Other vasodilatory medications such as minoxidil, nitrates, and hydralazine
- Surgical renal sympathetic denervation, used with success in some patients with resistant hypertension

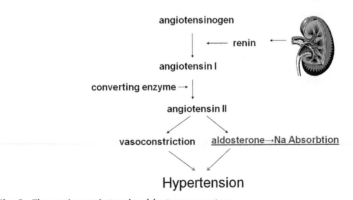

Fig. 2. The renin-angiotensin-aldosterone system.

SCREENING FOR HYPERTENSION DURING DENTAL VISITS

The dental visit provides an opportunity to screen large percentages of the population for hypertension. The Centers for Disease Control and Prevention (CDC) estimated that 65.4% of Americans older than 2 years had at least one dental visit in 2009.[12] Sproat and colleagues[13] noted that 59% of the population attends annual dental appointments in the United Kingdom, and Jontel and Glick[14] reported that 95% of the population in Sweden between the ages of 30 and 64 had used the Swedish dental health system within 5 years.

Screening for hypertension at dental office visits has been explored in multiple studies.[13–16] Fernandez-Feijoo and colleagues[15] screened 154 patients who presented for a dental checkup in Spain over a 6-month period in 2008. Forty-five of 154 (29.2%) patients had an SBP greater than 140 mm Hg and/or a DBP greater than 90 mm Hg, 33 of whom did not carry a diagnosis of hypertension before that visit. After referral to a physician, this screening resulted in 18 patients starting pharmacologic or nonpharmacologic therapy for hypertension.

Sproat and colleagues[13] screened patients older than 18 years for hypertension over a 3-day period at a dental practice in the United Kingdom, and found 44 of 144 (39%) of patients to have an SBP greater than 140 mm Hg and/or a DBP greater than 90 mm Hg. Thirty-six of these 44 patients (82%) had not been diagnosed with hypertension previously, and this increased blood pressure was not associated with increased anxiety as measured by the Dental Anxiety Scale (DAS).

Jontel and Glick[14] screened 200 patients with visits at 10 dental practices in Sweden for hypertension, hyperlipidemia, and hyperglycemia, and used the Heart-Score scale to determine their cardiovascular risk. Twelve of 200 patients (6%) had a greater than 10% risk of a fatal cardiovascular event in the next 10 years based on this screening, ultimately resulting in 7 patients being treated medically for hypertension or hyperlipidemia.

Glick and colleagues[16] extracted data from the National Health and Nutrition Examination Survey (NHANES) database. These investigators examined patients aged 45 to 85 years with no specific risk factor for coronary heart disease, who had seen a dentist in the last year but who had not seen a physician during that time. Eighteen percent of males in this population had a >10% Framingham risk for experiencing a coronary heart disease event within 10 years.

These studies demonstrate that screening for hypertension at dental visits allows for the identification of patients with previously undiagnosed hypertension, poorly controlled hypertension, and patients at increased risk for cardiovascular events. It is because of this opportunity and the relative ease of conducting blood pressure screening that many experts have agreed with the JNC 7 in recommending screening for hypertension at dental office visits.[13–15,17–19] Measurement of blood pressure should be done in the dental office at regular intervals.

HYPERTENSIVE MEDICATIONS AND DENTAL CARE
Blood Pressure Readings that Contraindicate Dental Care

No studies to date have associated hypertension at dental visits with adverse dental or cardiovascular outcomes. Many practitioners a SBP less than 180 or a DBP less than 110 mm Hg as the cutoff for performing urgent procedures without medical consultation.[17] Asymptomatic patients with blood pressures lower than these parameters are considered to be safe to undergo urgent and elective dental procedures.

It is important for dentists to recognize when hypertension can be acutely dangerous. This condition, known as hypertensive emergency, exists when a patient is exhibiting end-organ effects of severe hypertension and the SBP is greater than 180 or the DBP is less than 120 mm Hg. The organs that may be affected by such elevations, and the symptoms that a patient may have as a result of these effects, are shown in **Table 4**. Patients with severe hypertension and without these symptoms can be referred for urgent medical referral as an outpatient, whereas patients with these symptoms should be immediately referred to the emergency department.

Side Effects of Antihypertensive Medications

Oral and dental complaints are common in patients taking medications for hypertension. One study concluded that oral abnormality or complaints were found in 14% of patients attending a cardiology clinic who were taking antihypertensive medications.[20] Dentists should also be aware of other relevant side effects of these medications. A review of some of the most pertinent side effects of blood pressure medications for dentists (**Table 5**) follows.

Oral/dental side effects

Dry mouth (xerostomia) and dental caries Dry mouth is the most commonly reported oral side effect of antihypertensive medications.[20] It has been reported as a side effect in more than 10% of patients who take ACEIs, thiazide diuretics, loop diuretics, and clonidine.[21] For example, dry mouth has been reported in between 4.9% and 67% of patients taking clonidine, a central-acting α-blocker.[22–24] Xerostomia, in turn, increases the risk for dental caries,[21] and although a direct relationship has not been established, patients taking antihypertensive medications may be at increased risk of root decay.[25] The mechanism for xerostomia may be via direct action of medications on the salivary gland, resulting in decreased salivation. This effect may be dose dependent.[24,26]

Treatment of dry mouth may involve changing offending medications if possible. The use of parasympathomimetic medications such as pilocarpine is common, as are the recommendations of frequent sips of water, the use of sugarless candy or gum, minimizing caffeine intake, and avoiding the use of alcohol-containing mouthwashes.[17]

Gingival hyperplasia Calcium-channel blockers are commonly used medications in the treatment of hypertension, the 2 categories of which are dihydropyridines (peripheral-acting medications such as nifedipine and amlodipine) and nondihydropyridines (central-acting medications such as verapamil and diltiazem). Although more commonly observed with the use of dihydropyridines, drug-induced gingival overgrowth (DIGO) has been reported as a side effect of both classes of calcium-channel blockers with an incidence that has been reported from 6% to 83%.[27–33] This effect may be dose dependent (**Fig. 3**).

Risk factors for the development of DIGO include increased plaque-related gingival inflammation and the use of other drugs that cause gingival hyperplasia (ie,

Table 4	
Symptoms of hypertensive emergency	
Affected Organ	**Symptoms**
Central nervous system	Headache, changes in vision, nausea, vomiting, changes in sensation, muscle weakness, slurred speech
Heart	Chest pain, shortness of breath
Eyes	Changes in vision
Kidneys	Blood in the urine

Table 5
Adverse events associated with antihypertensive medications, and management of these side effects

Adverse Event	Medication(s)	Treatment/Management
Xerostomia (dry mouth), dental caries	ACEIs Thiazides Loop diuretics Clonidine	Change offending medication Pilocarpine Frequent sips of water Sugarless candy/gum Minimize caffeine intake Minimize use of alcohol-containing mouthwashes
Gingival hyperplasia	Dihydropyridine CCBs Nondihydropyridine CCBs	Gingival surgery
Orthostatic hypotension	Multiple classes of antihypertensive medications	Patient should sit upright for a few minutes after a dental procedure before standing up
Dysguesia	ACEI, β-Blockers Acetazolamide Diltiazem	Change offending medication
Lichenoid reactions	Captopril Methyldopa Furosemide β-Blockers Thiazides NSAIDs (naproxen)[a]	Change offending medication Topical corticosteroids

Abbreviations: ACEI, angiotensin-converting enzyme inhibitor; CCB, calcium-channel blocker; NSAID, nonsteroidal anti-inflammatory drug.
[a] NSAIDs are not prescribed to treat hypertension, but are commonly used and are included in this table because of their association with lichenoid reactions.

cyclosporine, phenytoin). Histopathologically there is overgrowth or expanded connective tissue with inflammation, and an enlarged gingival epithelium.[34]

Most studies involving DIGO have involved patients who were taking cyclosporine after organ transplantation. These studies suggest that DIGO be prevented with the

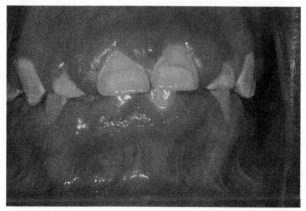

Fig. 3. Nifedipine-induced gingival hyperplasia, demonstrating enlargement of the interdental papillae and partial coverage of the crowns of the teeth. (*Courtesy of* Dr Ira B. Lamster, Columbia University College of Dental Medicine.)

use of oral-hygiene regimens initiated when the medication regimen is started.[35] This approach is intended to decrease the plaque-induced inflammation that may be a significant contributor to DIGO. Chlorhexidine rinses, folic acid rinses, and antibiotics have also been used in some cases but are not generally recommended. Gingival surgery is the most effective treatment of DIGO, but recurrence is common.[35]

Dysguesia (taste alteration) Dysguesia has been reported in the use of many medications, including antihypertensive medications such as β-blockers, acetazolamide, diltiazem, and ACEls. It has been postulated that dysguesia may result through a mechanism affecting salivary handling of metal ions such as magnesium.[36,37]

Lichenoid reactions Lichenoid reactions, particularly lichen planus, have been reported in patients taking antihypertensive medications including captopril, methyldopa, furosemide, β-blockers, and thiazides.[38,39] Oral lichen planus has also been reported in patients who have used nonsteroidal anti-inflammatory drugs (NSAIDs),[40] particularly naproxen.[41] The pathophysiologic mechanism of how these medications cause such dermatologic effects is not clear. The lichenoid reaction will often resolve after discontinuation of the offending medication. Topical corticosteroids may be used if the medication must be continued or if the lesions persist.[17]

Other relevant side effects

Orthostatic hypotension Orthostatic hypotension (OH) is defined as a decrease in SBP of at least 20 mm Hg or DBP of 10 mm Hg within 3 minutes of standing.[42] A patient with OH may experience light-headedness or syncope. OH results from the inability of the autonomic nervous system to achieve adequate blood return to the heart and appropriate vasoconstriction to maintain blood pressure and cerebral perfusion. OH may be caused by antihypertensive medications that affect the autonomic nervous system (clonidine and β-blockers), medications that cause vasodilation (terazosin, hydralazine, calcium-channel blockers), and those that cause volume depletion (diuretics).

Dentists may avoid OH by asking patients who are taking antihypertensive medications to sit upright for a few minutes before standing after undergoing evaluations and procedures.

Blood Pressure Effects of Medications Commonly Used During Dental Procedures

Vasoconstrictors: epinephrine

Vasoconstrictors are used in combination with local anesthetics such as lidocaine during dental procedures to decrease systemic toxicity, increase the duration and effectiveness of anesthesia, and provide hemostasis during surgery.[43] A commonly used cartridge in the United States contains 1.8 mL of 2% lidocaine with 1:100,000 epinephrine, for a total of 18 µg of epinephrine per cartridge. Epinephrine stimulates both α- and β-receptors on multiple tissues throughout the body, and its cardiovascular effects when used during dental procedures have been explored in many studies.

Local oral anesthesia with epinephrine has been shown to increase circulating plasma levels of epinephrine. Knoll-Kohler and colleagues[44] showed that plasma levels of epinephrine, as well as heart rate, increased in young, healthy subjects who had received lidocaine with 20 or 80 µg of epinephrine. This effect seemed to be dose dependent. Of interest, the heart rate increased and the DBP and mean blood pressure both decreased with the use of epinephrine. This effect on increased heart rate and decreased blood pressure has been attributed to β2-receptor stimulation in myocytes and arterioles.[18] Similarly, Dionne and colleagues[43] explored the cardiovascular effects of lidocaine with or without 54 µg of epinephrine during tooth extraction. Plasma epinephrine levels increased greater than 200% in the epinephrine group compared with control. Heart rate increased regardless of inclusion of epinephrine, and this effect was attenuated by preprocedure administration of the benzodiazepine diazepam. Bader and colleagues[45] reviewed the literature for cardiovascular effects in hypertensive patients undergoing dental procedures and who used anesthesia with and without epinephrine. Although the data were limited (only 6 studies were deemed to be acceptable for inclusion), the investigators concluded that the risk for cardiovascular events is low in this patient population despite occasional case reports of adverse reactions with the use of antihypertensive medications, which may interact with epinephrine at doses of 1 to 3 cartridges.

Further studies have been conducted using epinephrine-containing anesthesia in groups at higher risk for cardiovascular events, including patients with coronary artery disease,[46,47] valvular disease,[48] and heart transplants[49,50]; other vasoconstrictive agents have been used with success outside the United States in patients at high risk for ventricular arrhythmias.[50] Although Conrado and colleagues[46] found evidence of cardiac ischemia in the group receiving epinephrine, and Meechan and colleagues[49] found an increased heart rate without elevated blood pressure or clinical events in heart transplant recipients undergoing dental procedures with lidocaine and 55 µg of epinephrine, these data have not been replicated. The rate of adverse reactions remains low enough such that a recommendation against the use of epinephrine-containing anesthetic solutions, even in these high-risk populations, cannot be made.

One possible confounder is the effect of pain and/or anxiety on hemodynamics during dental office visits. Silvestre and colleagues[51] measured blood pressure during tooth extractions in patients without hypertension who received anesthesia with and without epinephrine, and observed an increase in blood pressure in both groups that did not differ significantly from each another. This elevated blood pressure was attributed to anxiety regarding the procedure. The same investigators studied patients with controlled "mild to moderate hypertension" (<139/89 mm Hg) who were undergoing tooth extraction with 1 to 3 cartridges of anesthetic with or without 4% epinephrine, and found only an increase in the SBP of patients who did not receive epinephrine.[52]

The cardiovascular effects of epinephrine used during dental procedures may be potentiated by the use of medications such as tricyclic antidepressants (such as imipramine and amitriptyline), nonselective β-blockers (such as propranolol and nadolol), and general anesthetics (halothane and thiopental). In settings where these medications are in use or administered, some experts recommend decreasing the dose and increasing the time interval between epinephrine injections.[53]

Epinephrine is present in higher dosages in the epinephrine-impregnated gingival retraction cords used when taking an impression for a crown. The amount of epinephrine in one retraction cord may be equivalent to 12 standard cartridges, and therefore has a higher theoretical risk of adverse cardiovascular events.[54] Hatch and colleagues[54] demonstrated that the use of epinephrine-containing retraction cords led to a significant increase in plasma catecholamines, but not in heart rate or blood pressure, in 9 healthy subjects (with intact gingival crevices) compared with retraction cords that did not contain epinephrine. Further studies have shown that circulating epinephrine levels are even higher with the use these retraction cords with a disrupted gingival crevice.[55] One death has been reported in the setting of the use of epinephrine-containing gingival retraction cords.[56] The patient was a healthy 36-year-old man who had ventricular fibrillation and a cardiac arrest while undergoing extensive dental restoration procedures using an epinephrine-containing retraction cord and general anesthesia with halothane.[56]

Dentists should be aware of the physiology of epinephrine, its pharmacokinetics, potential side effects, and medication interactions. When used in doses of 1 to 3 cartridges (18–54 μg), epinephrine has not been associated with adverse cardiovascular outcomes and therefore should be considered safe to use in the absence of a contraindication. Moreover, dentists should be aware of the risk of high doses of epinephrine with gingival retraction cords, particularly in high-risk patients and with the use of medications that may potentiate the effects of epinephrine. In these settings, decreasing the dose of epinephrine administered, increasing the time interval between epinephrine injections, and using retraction cords that do not contain epinephrine should be considered.

Nonsteroidal anti-inflammatory drugs

NSAIDs are widely available medications both over the counter and by prescription, and are commonly used for both acute and chronic pain, including dental pain. Many studies and meta-analyses have shown that NSAIDs increase blood pressure, most significantly in those who have a diagnosis of hypertension.[57] Therefore it is important for dentists to ask their patients about NSAID use and to report this information to physicians if there is concern for chronic NSAID use, which may be a modifiable contributor to a patient's hypertension.

SUMMARY

Hypertension is the most commonly diagnosed disease worldwide, and is associated with increased cardiovascular risk and mortality. Many patients with hypertension have uncontrolled disease. The dental visit presents a unique opportunity to screen patients for undiagnosed and undertreated hypertension, which may lead to improved monitoring and treatment. Although there are no clinical studies, it is generally recommended that nonemergent procedures be avoided in patients with a blood pressure of greater than 180/110 mm Hg. Because of the high prevalence of disease and medication use for hypertension, dentists should be aware of the oral side effects of antihypertensive medications as well as the cardiovascular effects of medications commonly used during dental visits.

REFERENCES

1. Chobanian AV, Bakris GL, Black HR, et al. The Seventh Report of the Joint National Committee on Prevention, detection, evaluation, and treatment of high blood pressure: the JNC 7 report. JAMA 2003;289(19):2560–72.
2. Lewington S, Clarke R, Qizilbash N, et al. Age-specific relevance of usual blood pressure to vascular mortality: a meta-analysis of individual data for one million adults in 61 prospective studies. Lancet 2002;360(9349):1903–13.
3. Neal B, MacMahon S, Chapman N. Effects of ACE inhibitors, calcium antagonists, and other blood-pressure-lowering drugs: results of prospectively designed overviews of randomised trials. Blood Pressure Lowering Treatment Trialists' Collaboration. Lancet 2000;356(9246):1955–64.
4. Smulyan H, Mukherjee R, Sheehe PR, et al. Cuff and aortic pressure differences during dobutamine infusion: a study of the effects of systolic blood pressure amplification. Am Heart J 2010;159(3):399–405.
5. Verdecchia P. Prognostic value of ambulatory blood pressure: current evidence and clinical implications. Hypertension 2000;35(3):844–51.
6. Pickering TG, James GD, Boddie C, et al. How common is white coat hypertension? JAMA 1988;259(2):225–8.

7. Gustavsen PH, Hoegholm A, Bang LE, et al. White coat hypertension is a cardiovascular risk factor: a 10-year follow-up study. J Hum Hypertens 2003;17(12):811–7.
8. Mann SJ. Drug therapy for resistant hypertension: simplifying the approach. J Clin Hypertens (Greenwich) 2011;13(2):120–30.
9. Chobanian AV, Hill M. National Heart, Lung, and Blood Institute workshop on sodium and blood pressure: a critical review of current scientific evidence. Hypertension 2000;35(4):858–63.
10. Kooman JP, van der Sande FM, Leunissen KM. Sodium, blood pressure and cardiovascular pathology: is it all volaemia? Nephrol Dial Transplant 2004;19(5):1046–9.
11. Appel LJ, Moore TJ, Obarzanek E, et al. A clinical trial of the effects of dietary patterns on blood pressure. DASH Collaborative Research Group. N Engl J Med 1997;336(16):1117–24.
12. Health, United States, 2010, with special feature on death and dying. 2011. Available at: http://www.cdc.gov/nchs/data/hus/hus10.pdf. Accessed March 1, 2012.
13. Sproat C, Beheshti S, Harwood AN, et al. Should we screen for hypertension in general dental practice? Br Dent J 2009;207(6):275–7.
14. Jontell M, Glick M. Oral health care professionals' identification of cardiovascular disease risk among patients in private dental offices in Sweden. J Am Dent Assoc 2009;140(11):1385–91.
15. Fernandez-Feijoo J, Nunez-Orjales JL, Limeres-Posse J, et al. Screening for hypertension in a primary care dental clinic. Med Oral Patol Oral Cir Bucal 2010;15(3):e467–72.
16. Glick M, Greenberg BL. The potential role of dentists in identifying patients' risk of experiencing coronary heart disease events. J Am Dent Assoc 2005;136(11):1541–6.
17. Herman WW, Konzelman JL Jr, Prisant LM. New national guidelines on hypertension: a summary for dentistry. J Am Dent Assoc 2004;135(5):576–84 [quiz: 653–4].
18. Little JW. The impact on dentistry of recent advances in the management of hypertension. Oral Surg Oral Med Oral Pathol Oral Radiol Endod 2000;90(5):591–9.
19. Muzyka BC, Glick M. The hypertensive dental patient. J Am Dent Assoc 1997;128(8):1109–20.
20. Habbab KM, Moles DR, Porter SR. Potential oral manifestations of cardiovascular drugs. Oral Dis 2010;16(8):769–73.
21. Guggenheimer J, Moore PA. Xerostomia: etiology, recognition and treatment. J Am Dent Assoc 2003;134(1):61–9 [quiz: 118–9].
22. Wing LM, Reid JL, Davies DS, et al. Pharmacokinetic and concentration-effect relationships of clonidine in essential hypertension. Eur J Clin Pharmacol 1977;12(6):463–9.
23. Breidthardt J, Schumacher H, Mehlburger L. Long-term (5 year) experience with transdermal clonidine in the treatment of mild to moderate hypertension. Clin Auton Res 1993;3(6):385–90.
24. Jaattela A. Comparison of guanfacine and clonidine as antihypertensive agents. Br J Clin Pharmacol 1980;10(Suppl 1):67S–70S.
25. Streckfus CF, Strahl RC, Welsh S. Anti-hypertension medications: an epidemiological factor in the prevalence of root decay among geriatric patients suffering from hypertension. Clin Prev Dent 1990;12(3):26–9.
26. Watson GE, Pearson SK, Bowen WH. The effect of chronic clonidine administration on salivary glands and caries in the rat. Caries Res 2000;34(2):194–200.
27. Ellis JS, Seymour RA, Steele JG, et al. Prevalence of gingival overgrowth induced by calcium channel blockers: a community-based study. J Periodontol 1999;70(1):63–7.

28. Kaur G, Verhamme KM, Dieleman JP, et al. Association between calcium channel blockers and gingival hyperplasia. J Clin Periodontol 2010;37(7):625–30.
29. Barak S, Engelberg IS, Hiss J. Gingival hyperplasia caused by nifedipine. Histopathologic findings. J Periodontol 1987;58(9):639–42.
30. Tagawa T, Nakamura H, Murata M. Marked gingival hyperplasia induced by nifedipine. Int J Oral Maxillofac Surg 1990;19(2):72–3.
31. Akimoto Y, Tanaka S, Omata H, et al. Gingival hyperplasia induced by nifedipine. J Nihon Univ Sch Dent 1991;33(3):174–81.
32. Fattore L, Stablein M, Bredfeldt G, et al. Gingival hyperplasia: a side effect of nifedipine and diltiazem. Spec Care Dentist 1991;11(3):107–9.
33. Burkes EJ Jr, Jacoway JR, Stevens DT, et al. Nifedipine-induced gingival hyperplasia. J Tenn Dent Assoc 1992;72(2):35–7.
34. Seymour RA. Effects of medications on the periodontal tissues in health and disease. Periodontol 2000 2006;40:120–9.
35. Mavrogiannis M, Ellis JS, Thomason JM, et al. The management of drug-induced gingival overgrowth. J Clin Periodontol 2006;33(6):434–9.
36. Ackerman BH, Kasbekar N. Disturbances of taste and smell induced by drugs. Pharmacotherapy 1997;17(3):482–96.
37. Musumeci V, Di Salvo S, Zappacosta B, et al. Salivary electrolytes in treated hypertensives at low or normal sodium diet. Clin Exp Hypertens 1993;15(2):245–56.
38. Ciancio SG. Medications' impact on oral health. J Am Dent Assoc 2004;135(10):1440–8 [quiz: 1468–9].
39. Ellgehausen P, Elsner P, Burg G. Drug-induced lichen planus. Clin Dermatol 1998;16(3):325–32.
40. Potts AJ, Hamburger J, Scully C. The medication of patients with oral lichen planus and the association of nonsteroidal anti-inflammatory drugs with erosive lesions. Oral Surg Oral Med Oral Pathol 1987;64(5):541–3.
41. Gunes AT, Fetil E, Ilknur T, et al. Naproxen-induced lichen planus: report of 55 cases. Int J Dermatol 2006;45(6):709–12.
42. Medow MS, Stewart JM, Sanyal S, et al. Pathophysiology, diagnosis, and treatment of orthostatic hypotension and vasovagal syncope. Cardiol Rev 2008;16(1):4–20.
43. Dionne RA, Goldstein DS, Wirdzek PR. Effects of diazepam premedication and epinephrine-containing local anesthetic on cardiovascular and plasma catecholamine responses to oral surgery. Anesth Analg 1984;63(7):640–6.
44. Knoll-Kohler E, Frie A, Becker J, et al. Changes in plasma epinephrine concentration after dental infiltration anesthesia with different doses of epinephrine. J Dent Res 1989;68(6):1098–101.
45. Bader JD, Bonito AJ, Shugars DA. A systematic review of cardiovascular effects of epinephrine on hypertensive dental patients. Oral Surg Oral Med Oral Pathol Oral Radiol Endod 2002;93(6):647–53.
46. Conrado VC, de Andrade J, de Angelis GA, et al. Cardiovascular effects of local anesthesia with vasoconstrictor during dental extraction in coronary patients. Arq Bras Cardiol 2007;88(5):507–13.
47. Vanderheyden PJ, Williams RA, Sims TN. Assessment of ST segment depression in patients with cardiac disease after local anesthesia. J Am Dent Assoc 1989;119(3):407–12.
48. Laragnoit AB, Neves RS, Neves IL, et al. Locoregional anesthesia for dental treatment in cardiac patients: a comparative study of 2% plain lidocaine and 2% lidocaine with epinephrine (1:100,000). Clinics (Sao Paulo) 2009;64(3):177–82.

49. Meechan JG, Parry G, Rattray DT, et al. Effects of dental local anaesthetics in cardiac transplant recipients. Br Dent J 2002;192(3):161–3.
50. Borea G, Montebugnoli L, Capuzzi P, et al. Circulatory dynamics during dental operations in patients with heart transplants. Quintessence Int 1993;24(10): 749–51.
51. Silvestre FJ, Verdu MJ, Sanchis JM, et al. Effects of vasoconstrictors in dentistry upon systolic and diastolic arterial pressure. Med Oral 2001;6(1):57–63.
52. Silvestre FJ, Salvador-Martinez I, Bautista D, et al. Clinical study of hemodynamic changes during extraction in controlled hypertensive patients. Med Oral Patol Oral Cir Bucal 2011;16(3):e354–8.
53. Yagiela JA. Adverse drug interactions in dental practice: interactions associated with vasoconstrictors. Part V of a series. J Am Dent Assoc 1999;130(5):701–9.
54. Hatch CL, Chernow B, Terezhalmy GT, et al. Plasma catecholamine and hemodynamic responses to the placement of epinephrine-impregnated gingival retraction cord. Oral Surg Oral Med Oral Pathol 1984;58(5):540–4.
55. Shaw DH, Krejci RF, Todd GL, et al. Determination of plasma catecholamines in dogs after experimental gingival retraction with epinephrine-impregnated cord. Arch Oral Biol 1987;32(3):217–9.
56. Hilley MD, Milam SB, Giescke AH Jr, et al. Fatality associated with the combined use of halothane and gingival retraction cord. Anesthesiology 1984;60(6):587–8.
57. Frishman WH. Effects of nonsteroidal anti-inflammatory drug therapy on blood pressure and peripheral edema. Am J Cardiol 2002;89(6A):18D–25D.

Tobacco Cessation in the Dental Office

David Albert, DDS, MPH*, Angela Ward, RDH, MA

KEYWORDS

- Tobacco cessation • Pharmacotherapeutics • Oral pathology • Addiction

KEY POINTS

- Evidence based tobacco-cessation guidelines (the 5 A's: Ask, Advise, Assess, Assist, and Arrange) when used by clinicians are effective in reducing tobacco use and obtaining successful quits by patients.
- Numerous investigations involving dentists have provided evidence that counseling by clinicians with regard to the 5 A's can be achieved.
- Dentists have been encouraged by organizations including the American Dental Association, the Centers for Disease Control and Prevention, and the US Public Health Service to provide instruction and intervention on tobacco cessation in the dental office. The dental provider is in the unique position to relate oral findings to the patient and to provide advice to tobacco-using patients about quitting the habit.
- Dentists are in a position where they are able to assess patients' self-addiction, and level of readiness to quit tobacco use. With this information, dentists then can provide assistance with the quit by providing an appropriate pharmacotherapeutic aid to help patients stop using tobacco, and thereby improve their oral and overall health.

INTRODUCTION

Tobacco use is the principal cause of preventable disease and death in the United States. One in 2 long-term smokers will die of a tobacco-related illness.[1] In annual estimates, smoking accounts for 438,000 premature deaths among smokers and an additional 38,000 deaths in nonsmokers from the effects of second-hand smoke.[2]

Seventy percent of those who smoke want to quit and approximately 41% try to quit each year.[3] However, despite the availability of a wide array of effective smoking cessation treatments, more than 60% will try to quit without assistance. Unfortunately for those smokers who try to quit alone, fewer than 5% will still be abstinent at 1 year.[4] A dentist's advice to quit coupled with pharmacotherapy can double or triple success rates.[5] Dentists are in an ideal position to offer smoking interventions, as 65% of adults 18 years and older visit the dentist annually. Approximately 50% of smokers visit

Division of Community Health, Section of Social and Behavioral Sciences, Columbia University College of Dental Medicine, 630 West 168th Street, New York, NY 10032, USA
* Corresponding author.
E-mail address: daa1@columbia.edu

Dent Clin N Am 56 (2012) 747–770
http://dx.doi.org/10.1016/j.cden.2012.07.004
0011-8532/12/$ – see front matter © 2012 Elsevier Inc. All rights reserved.

dental.theclinics.com

a dentist within any year,[6] allowing dentists the opportunity to discuss tobacco use, its visible oral consequences, and cessation.

The risks of smoking can be reduced by successfully quitting at any age. Quitting smoking has immediate as well as long-term benefits, reducing risks for diseases caused by smoking and improving health in general. Quitting smoking immediately reduces risks for cardiovascular disease and cancer. For example, the risk of myocardial infarction decreases by 50% within the first year of abstinence.[7] Smoking cessation also reduces risk for low birth weight, respiratory illness, and sudden infant death syndrome (SIDS) among the children of smokers.[8] Smokers who stop smoking even at the age of 40 or 50 years avoid more than 90% of the risk of lung cancer associated with tobacco.[9]

Indirect exposure to tobacco smoke is also an important risk factor for premature death and disease in children and adults who do not smoke. The 2006 Surgeon General Report on the health consequences of involuntary exposure to tobacco smoke concluded that there is no risk-free level of exposure to second-hand smoke (SHS).[8] Children exposed are at increased risk for SIDS, acute respiratory infections, ear problems, and more severe asthma.[8] Exposure of adults to SHS has immediate adverse effects on the cardiovascular system, and causes coronary heart disease and lung cancer.[10] It is therefore equally important to inquire about exposure to SHS at home and to recommend that patients create a smoke-free home to protect children and nonsmoking adults.

Smokeless tobacco products, which consist of chewing tobacco and moist and dry snuff, have been used for thousands of years especially among populations in South America and Southeast Asia. However, these products have gained worldwide popularity including in the United States. Smokeless tobacco use is not a safe alternative for smoking, and can lead to nicotine addiction and dependence similar to that produced by cigarette smoking. There is sufficient evidence that the use of smokeless tobacco causes cancer in humans. Smokeless tobacco, like smoked tobacco, contains carcinogens, which contribute to cancers of the oral cavity and pharynx and increase the risk of other head and neck cancers.[11] Smokeless tobacco use also causes several noncancerous oral conditions, such as leukoplakia, gingival recession, alveolar bone loss, and caries.

An analysis of long-term national trends in smokeless tobacco use reported that considerable progress has been made in reducing adult and adolescent smokeless tobacco use.[12] Smokeless tobacco use has declined among the young, with a decrease noted particularly among boys in most subpopulations in all grades. The largest decline was noted among adolescent males.[12] Among adult men significant declines in smokeless tobacco use was also noted for all age groups, except for men aged 25 to 44 years.[12] Men within this age group now have the highest prevalence of smokeless tobacco use among all adult age groups.[12]

PERIODONTAL DISEASE

Cigarette smoking can lead to periodontitis and the loss of alveolar bone support (**Fig. 1**).[13]

A plethora of substances associated with cigarette smoking have the potential to adversely affect health. These substances include nicotine, which undergoes tissue absorption and enters the bloodstream at a level of 2 to 3 mg per cigarette, and several gases (notably carbon monoxide and hydrogen cyanide) that are inhaled at an approximate volume of 20 to 30 mL per cigarette.[14] These toxic substances have a multitude of biologically plausible effects, including vasoconstriction resulting in tissue ischemia,

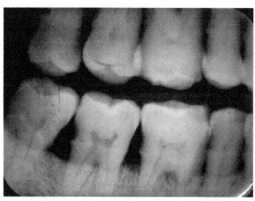

Fig. 1. Tobacco use and periodontal disease. (*Courtesy of* David A. Albert, DDS, MPH, Columbia University College of Dental Medicine.)

impaired inflammatory vascular response, impaired oxygen metabolism, impaired polymorphonuclear leukocyte chemotaxis, deficient phagocytosis, and cellular repair. Direct damage to macrophages and fibroblasts has also been reported to occur, resulting in delayed wound healing.

The gingival tissues of smokers are known to exhibit increased keratinization, which obscures the signs of gingival inflammation and suppresses the occurrence of bleeding on probing. Despite this misleading clinical appearance, multiple epidemiologic studies have unequivocally demonstrated that the prevalence of periodontitis, expressed as loss of clinical attachment or radiographic loss of alveolar bone support, is higher in smokers than in nonsmokers.[14] Of importance, the difference in prevalence persists after adjustments for age, gender, race, educational level, and oral hygiene practices. In addition, studies have shown that smoking may alter the composition of the subgingival microbiota, and a higher level of colonization by pathogenic bacteria (notably *Porphyromonas gingivalis* and *Bacteroides forsythus*) has been shown to occur in shallow sites of smokers when compared with clinically similar sites in nonsmokers.

Longitudinal studies of both treated and untreated periodontitis have demonstrated higher progression of attachment loss or bone loss in smokers than in nonsmokers.[15] A dose-response relationship between exposure to smoking, measured in "pack years," and extent and severity of progressive periodontitis has been demonstrated as well.

Treatment studies have provided additional insights on the detrimental role of smoking on periodontal health.[16] The vast majority of patients who do not respond well to periodontal therapy, the so-called refractory patients, are smokers.[17] Overall, smokers show a less favorable response than nonsmokers to conventional periodontal therapy. The difference in response becomes particularly pronounced in more elaborate treatment procedures, such as regenerative periodontal therapies (guided tissue regeneration and grafting procedures), which have been shown to be significantly less successful and predictable in smokers.[18]

Studies have demonstrated the beneficial effects of smoking cessation on periodontal health. Progression of bone loss was decreased in patients who quit smoking in comparison with subjects who continued to smoke throughout the observation period.[19] Similar positive effects of smoking cessation have been observed in prospective studies studying tooth loss. Indeed, the rate of tooth loss was significantly decreased in subjects who quit smoking.

Cigarette smoking is one of the most important risk factors for periodontitis, as it fulfills all of the stipulated epidemiologic criteria required to impute a causative relationship. Studies have calculated that a substantial percentage of the variance of periodontitis in the population (as high as 50%) can be attributed to smoking alone.[20] Behavioral scientists have suggested that dentists are probably the best-suited health care professionals to both serve as patient educators on the adverse effects of smoking on oral and systemic health, and to implement smoking cessation. Dentists must therefore expand their preventive and therapeutic armamentarium to include strategies on smoking cessation.

DENTAL CARIES

The link between dental caries and tobacco is not conclusive. Smokeless tobacco can contribute to increased acid attack on the enamel surface if the brand of tobacco contains high concentrations of sugar. Gingival recession often occurs at the location the user habitually places smokeless tobacco. This recession exposes cementum to plaque and subsequently to reduction in pH from acids produced by cariogenic bacteria metabolizing sugars. There may therefore be a higher incidence of cervical or root caries in smokeless tobacco users (**Fig. 2**).[21]

AESTHETICS

Cosmetic conditions such as tobacco stains are difficult to treat successfully. Tobacco stains can penetrate into enamel and restorative materials, creating brown to yellow darkening of teeth, discoloration of nonmetallic restorations, and dark outlines around restorative margins. Tobacco staining of removable prosthetic appliances can be a problem; patients are frequently unable to remove tenacious stains with denture cleaners and may become dissatisfied with their appliance and appearance (**Fig. 3**).

The use of smokeless tobacco often results in severe abrasion and subsequent exposure of dentin that becomes stained (**Fig. 4**).[22] Abrasives contained in chewing tobacco can wear away considerable portions of the occluding surfaces of teeth.

The ever increasing demand for cosmetic bleaching may be associated with tobacco use. Good results with over-the-counter whitening systems, office-based bleaching systems, or with lasers may be difficult to achieve if a patient is a heavy tobacco user. Repeated treatments, or increased length of time that may be needed for deep stains, can result in increased sensitivity.

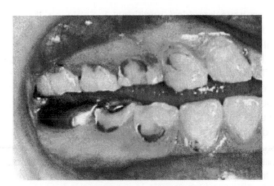

Fig. 2. Smokeless tobacco user with recession and cervical caries lesions. (*Courtesy of* Murray Bartley, DDS, Oregon Health & Sciences University, School of Dentistry.)

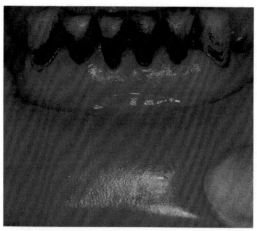

Fig. 3. Tobacco stains. (*From* Mecklenburg RE, Greenspan D, Kleinman DV, et al. Tobacco effects in the mouth: a National Cancer Institute and National Institute of Dental Research Guide for Health Professionals. Bethesda (MD): United States Department of Health and Human Services, Public Health Service, National Institutes of Health;1994. NIH Publication No. 94–3330.)

Bonding, or the placement of porcelain veneers, may be compromised if the patient continues to smoke during or after treatment. It is not unusual for these patients to have loss of attachment and recession, resulting in poor long-term aesthetics and the possible need for retreatment to achieve a better result.

Halitosis or bad breath is common in tobacco users. Tobacco users often chew gum or use sweetened candies to mask sulfurous smells present in their breath. If these patients opt for gums and breath mints that are sweetened with sugars, repeated drops in plaque pH occur, subjecting the user to increased acid attack and dental caries.

Hairy tongue (**Fig. 5**), an overgrowth of the filiform papillae of the tongue that can trap plaque and tobacco residues, contributes to poor appearance and bad breath.

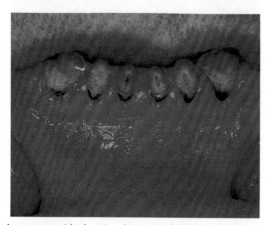

Fig. 4. Smokeless tobacco user with abrasion. (*From* Mecklenburg RE, Greenspan D, Kleinman DV, et al. Tobacco effects in the mouth: a National Cancer Institute and National Institute of Dental Research Guide for Health Professionals. Bethesda (MD): United States Department of Health and Human Services, Public Health Service, National Institutes of Health;1994. NIH Publication No. 94–3330.)

ORAL CANCER

Almost three-quarters of oral-cavity and pharyngeal cancers are linked to the use of smoked and smokeless tobacco.[23] Smoked and smokeless tobacco contains dangerous compounds, such as tar and nitrosamines, which have been linked with cancer. Smokeless tobacco users are prone to leukoplakia. The tongue is the most common site of oral cancer, and other cancer sites include the mouth, lips, throat, parts of the nose, and the larynx. Approximately 30,000 new cases of oral cancer are diagnosed in the United States each year, and about 9000 people die of the disease each year.[24] While oral cancer accounts for about 4% of all cancers diagnosed in the United States, the survival rate from oral cancer is among the lowest of those of major cancers.[25] Oral cancer includes a variety of lesions and tumors in and around the mouth, including cancers of the esophagus, larynx, and stomach.[25]

Excessive alcohol use is another risk factor. The combined use of alcohol and tobacco products poses a much greater risk than does either substance alone. Age is also a factor. Although it is possible to contract oral cancer at any age, more than 90% of oral cancers are diagnosed in people older than 40 years, with an average age at time of diagnosis of about 60 years.[24] Other factors that place a person at risk include viral infections, exposure to sunlight, and certain work-related exposures.

ORAL MUCOSAL LESIONS

Oral mucosal lesions occur more frequently in chronic tobacco users.[26] These lesions may occur because of carcinogens, toxins, and irritants that are present in tobacco. In addition, tobacco's drying effects, the exposure of oral tissues to heat from smoked tobacco, and the alteration in the oral pH can lead to an altered immune response

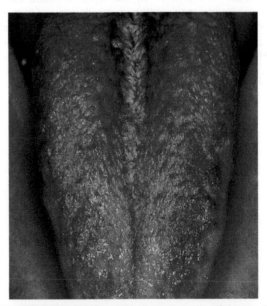

Fig. 5. Hairy tongue. (*From* Mecklenburg RE, Greenspan D, Kleinman DV, et al. Tobacco effects in the mouth: a National Cancer Institute and National Institute of Dental Research Guide for Health Professionals. Bethesda (MD): United States Department of Health and Human Services, Public Health Service, National Institutes of Health;1994. NIH Publication No. 94–3330.)

and a breakdown in the mucosal membrane that leads to increased exposure to viral and fungal infections.

LEUKOPLAKIA

Leukoplakia is defined as a white patch, or plaque, on the oral mucosa that cannot be classified clinically as any other disease. Tobacco use is the primary cause of leukoplakic lesions. Tobacco users are more likely than nonusers to have leukoplakia. The frequency and duration of tobacco use is directly related to the prevalence of leukoplakia.[26]

Smokeless tobacco placed in the mandibular anterior labial vestibule has produced characteristic alterations of oral mucosa. An extensive, white, slightly thickened plaque demonstrates a wrinkled, corrugated surface texture.

Snuff dipper's pouch may be a form of leukoplakia (**Fig. 6**). These white or red adherent lesions are tissue of various degrees of abnormal appearance, from white translucent patches to thickened, cracked areas. Although lesions can be found at any step of a continuous process, they are categorized into 3 degrees, with degree 3 being the most serious. However, lesions of any degree may convert to squamous cell carcinoma at a rate of 3% to 5%.[27]

NICOTINIC STOMATITIS

Nicotinic stomatitis appears as a diffuse palatal keratosis with chronic inflammation of the palatal salivary glands. It does not become malignant and is reversible with cessation of tobacco use.[26]

SMOKER'S MELANOSIS

Smoker's melanosis is a melanin pigmentation stimulated by smoking that may occur in the attached gingiva of about 5% to 10% of smokers.[28] It is more common in heavy smokers (**Fig. 7**).

TOBACCO CESSATION IN THE DENTAL OFFICE

When a smoker makes the decision to quit smoking, the assistance of a health care provider can be a critical aid to his or her success. Assisting patients in quitting

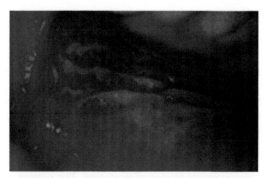

Fig. 6. Snuff dipper's pouch and leukoplakia. (*From* Mecklenburg RE, Greenspan D, Kleinman DV, et al. Tobacco effects in the mouth: a National Cancer Institute and National Institute of Dental Research Guide for Health Professionals. Bethesda (MD): United States Department of Health and Human Services, Public Health Service, National Institutes of Health;1994. NIH Publication No. 94–3330.)

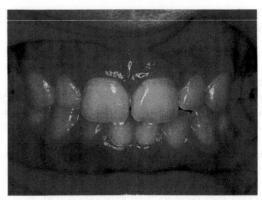

Fig. 7. Smoker's melanosis. (*From* Mecklenburg RE, Greenspan D, Kleinman DV, et al. Tobacco effects in the mouth: a National Cancer Institute and National Institute of Dental Research Guide for Health Professionals. Bethesda (MD): United States Department of Health and Human Services, Public Health Service, National Institutes of Health;1994. NIH Publication No. 94–3330.)

smoking can be done as part of a brief treatment or as part of an intensive treatment program. Studies have shown that when clinicians provide advice and brief assistance, patients are 2 times more likely to quit smoking compared with quitting on their own.[5] In addition, the use of cessation medication will enhance the clinician's advice and double the odds of quitting with advice alone.[5]

It is important to recognize that stopping tobacco use is a process and that there are several stages of quitting. When you work with tobacco-using patients, you will find them at varying degrees of readiness to make changes in their behavior. Some of the smokers you treat will be ready to take action, some may only be thinking about stopping, and others may be content with their smoking behavior.

The US Public Health Service recommends that dentists and dental hygienists be prepared to intervene with tobacco users who are willing to quit. The 5 major steps to intervention in the primary care setting, Ask, Advise, Assess, Assist, and Arrange (the 5 A's) are listed in **Table 1**. These intervention strategies are designed to be brief, requiring 3 minutes or less of direct clinician time at each encounter.[5]

THE 5 A'S
Ask

Before addressing a patient's tobacco use, the clinician should ask if he or she uses tobacco; this can be done by asking the patient directly when reviewing the patient's health history, or alternatively during the clinical examination. All it takes is 4 words, "Do you use tobacco?" Once it is established whether or not the patient uses tobacco, it is important to record the information in the patient's chart, thus making it easier to follow up when the patient returns for the next visit.

Advise

Clinicians should advise patients to quit at every visit. The patient should be urged to quit in a clear, strong, and personalized manner. In addition, the dental examination presents an opportunity to identify oral conditions related to tobacco use to the patient to increase the motivation to quit. Tobacco use contributes to periodontal disease, dental caries, aesthetic changes, oral cancer, and soft-tissue lesions.

Table 1 United States public health service 5A's for brief intervention	
The "5A's" for Brief Intervention	
Ask about tobacco use	Identify and document tobacco use status for every patient at every visit
Advise to quit	Urge every tobacco user to quit in a clear, strong, and personalized manner
Assess willingness to quit	Is the tobacco user willing to make a quit attempt at this time? If not, attempt to get him or her to consider quitting
Assist in quit attempt	Provide counseling and pharmacotherapy for patients interested in quitting
Arrange follow-up	Schedule follow-up visit to address successes, barriers, and the proper use and effectiveness of pharmacotherapy. It is preferable to schedule the first follow-up visit within a few days of any cessation attempt

Adapted from the U.S. Department of Health and Human Services June 2000 clinical practice guideline "treating tobacco use and dependence". To order the full guideline call 800-358-9295 or write: Publications Clearinghouse, P.O. Box 8547, Silver Spring, MD 20907. Also available on the Surgeon General's Web site: http://www.surgeongeneral.gov/tobacco/default.htm. Accessed May 7, 2012.

Assess

Clinicians often think that tobacco users do not want to discuss quitting. However, research has shown that the majority of smokers would like to quit. Even with patients who are not ready to quit using tobacco, it has been found that they are receptive to the clinician's advice. By getting patients to talk about their tobacco use, they may move closer to a decision to quit.

To focus your efforts on patients who are ready to make a change you will want to assess their readiness to quit at each appointment. Change does not progress in a straight line; people may seem disinterested about quitting, but may report an attempt to quit at their next visit. Or people may take action to quit, be unsuccessful, and become discouraged. Regular assessment at each visit is important.

The 0 to 10 quitting scale provides some insight into your patients' feelings about quitting and also provides you with the opportunity to continue your conversation on tobacco cessation by asking some follow-up questions. The goal is to engage your patients in talking and thinking about quitting, and gradually moving them from the lower part of the 0 to 10 scale, where they are not ready to quit, to the upper part, where they are ready to make an attempt to quit (**Fig. 8**).

Assist

When patients express an interest in quitting, clinicians should assist them by giving them information they can use that will help them quit. Clinicians can provide self-help materials and make referrals to local resources, and may also want to discuss the use of pharmacotherapy, such as nicotine gum or patches.

In addition to advice to quit and counseling, it is recommended that patients should be offered pharmacotherapy for tobacco cessation. Effective pharmacotherapy provides a 2- to 3-times higher cessation rate compared with placebo at any level of supportive care.[5] The goal of nicotine replacement therapy (NRT) is to safely replace the daily nicotine intake; about 1 mg of nicotine is absorbed per cigarette, hence a 1-pack-per-day (PPD) smoker requires replacement of approximately 20 mg of nicotine per day. Patients should continue with NRT until successful cessation and

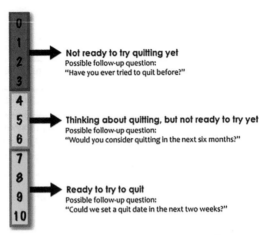

Fig. 8. Zero to 10 quitting scale. (*Courtesy of* Columbia Center for New Media Teaching and Learning; with permission.)

confidence in a smoke-free lifestyle has been achieved. Although this usually occurs after 8 to 12 weeks, some individuals may take longer, so a longer duration of therapy may be required, which is safe. Pharmacotherapies are not recommended for use in persons younger than 18 years or pregnant women.

Table 2 provides a quick reference guide for the dental clinician. For a more comprehensive listing of dosages, uses, contraindications, and adverse effects, please refer to the prescribing information provided by the manufacturer of the product, or the Physician Desk Reference.

Nicotine replacement therapy

The purpose of NRT is to safely replace an individual's daily nicotine intake that was obtained from tobacco use. A successful tobacco-cessation effort should adequately replace all the nicotine that is lost when a patient quits smoking. About 1 mg of nicotine is absorbed per cigarette; hence, a 1-PPD smoker requires replacement of approximately 20 mg of nicotine per day.

NRTs work by temporarily reducing symptoms of nicotine withdrawal after quitting smoking. NRTs are very safe when used as directed; there is little risk of your patient becoming dependent. With NRTs, blood concentrations of nicotine peak more slowly, reaching much lower levels in comparison with smoking. Your patient will not experience a nicotine "rush," but he or she also will not experience the painful cravings and withdrawal symptoms associated with quitting. NRTs help to take the edge off cigarette cravings without providing the tars and poisonous gases found in cigarettes.

Patients may prefer an NRT that offers self-administered dosing such as the gum, lozenge, or inhaler, because these options meet oral gratification needs and provide alternatives for patients at high risk for transdermal-related skin irritation. On the other hand, because the nicotine patch is worn continuously, it lessens chances of suffering from several of the major smoking withdrawal symptoms such as tenseness, irritability, drowsiness, and lack of concentration. The nasal spray reduces nicotine cravings within several minutes of dosing, and unlike the patch allows the user to self-dose as necessary. One should be aware, however, that the dependency potential is greater with the nicotine nasal spray than with other NRTs. In the dental office the NRTs are typically used as front-line pharmacotherapeutic aids. There are 5 types of NRTs: (1) over-the-counter NRTs including patch, gum, and lozenge, and (2) prescription NRTs including nasal spray and inhaler. The inhaler is infrequently used and is not covered in this article.

NRTs should not be used in patients with serious arrhythmias, or with severe or worsening angina. NRTs should be discontinued if tachycardia or palpitations occur. Do not use during the immediate postmyocardial infarction period. NRTs should be used with caution in patients with: (1) coronary heart disease, (2) vasospastic diseases, (3) hyperthyroidism, (4) pheochromocytoma, (5) insulin-dependent diabetes, (6) active peptic ulcer disease, (7) accelerated hypertension, and (8) bronchospastic disease. For comprehensive contraindications and adverse effects, refer to individual product inserts and to the Physician's Desk Reference (**Fig. 9**).

Nicotine gum Nicotine is bound to an ion-exchange resin and is added to a gum base. The nicotine from the gum is steadily released and then is absorbed via the blood vessels in the oral buccal mucosa. Some of the nicotine also goes into the saliva, and when swallowed, is absorbed through the gastrointestinal tract. Do not use in patients with poor dentition or complex fixed or removable dental prostheses.

Nicotine gum is available as 2 mg (use for <10 cigs/24 h or if patient smokes first cigarette within 30 minutes of waking up) and 4 mg (use for ≥10 cigs/24 h or if patient smokes first cigarette within 30 minutes of waking up). The dosage your patient will need is determined by how much he or she smokes. The 4-mg dose is suggested for most patients (even those smoking fewer than 10 cigarettes a day). Patient compliance with chewing (20–30 minutes per piece) and frequency of use are difficult to follow for the 2-mg dose.

For example, a 9-cigarettes-a-day smoker would need to replace 9 mg of nicotine. The recommended 2-mg dose would provide 1 mg of nicotine if chewed for 30 minutes. This patient would need to chew for 4.5 hours per day to replace all the nicotine present in the cigarettes, and this is difficult for most patients. Patients should not exceed 24 pieces of gum each day.

Dosage for nicotine gum:

1. Use 1 piece every 1 to 2 hours for the first 6 weeks or until the patient is comfortable with quit attempt
2. Use 1 piece every 2 to 4 hours for the next 3 weeks
3. Use 1 piece of gum every 4 to 8 hours for the next 3 weeks, until the patient gradually stops usage

Nicotine gum is not designed to be chewed like normal gum. It should be used in a "park and chew" way as follows: (1) insert a piece of gum into the mouth, (2) chew it a few times to break it down, until mouth "tingles", and (3) park it between the gum and cheek and leave it there. If the patient does not use the park and chew method and instead chews continuously without parking, the nicotine will be released directly into the saliva, swallowed, and absorbed through the gastrointestinal tract, resulting in severe nausea and tachycardia. Advise your patient not to eat or drink for 15 minutes before or while using the gum because this can reduce the absorption of the nicotine. Occasionally the gum may cause mild mucosal irritation. For comprehensive contraindications and adverse effects, refer to individual product inserts and to the Physician's Desk Reference.

Nicotine lozenge Nicotine is bound to an ion-exchange resin and is added to a sugar-free hard sweet lozenge. The nicotine from the lozenge is steadily released and then is absorbed via the blood vessels in the oral buccal mucosa. Some of the nicotine also goes into the saliva, is swallowed, and is absorbed through the

Table 2
Pharmacotherapy guide

Product	Best For	Precautions	Adverse Effects	Dosage	Tapering Schedule	Patient Education
Nicotine patch[a,b] 21 mg, 14 mg, 7 mg	For patients who smoke more than 10 cigarettes a day As an adjunctive medication in combination therapy treatment (with short-acting nicotine replacement therapies or Zyban)	Allergy to adhesive possible Serious arrhythmias or severe worsening angina Caution within 6 wk of myocardial infarction Discontinue if tachycardia or palpitations occur	Skin irritation or discoloration	≥10 cigs/24 h: 21 mg/24 h for 6 wk <10 cigs/24 h or <46 kg: 14 mg/24 h for 6 wk	≥10 cigs/24 h: 14 mg/24 h for 2 wk followed by 7 mg/24 h for 2 wk, then stop <10 cigs/24 h: 7 mg/24 h for 2 wk then stop	Apply daily to dry, hairless skin Focal rash common; rotate site daily Do not smoke while using these products
Nicotine gum[c] 4 mg, 2 mg	For patients who smoke less than one pack per day acceptable as solo therapy As an adjunctive medication in combination therapy treatment (with nicotine patch or Zyban)	Poor dentition May be inappropriate for use in patients with complete or large partial dentures Serious arrhythmias or severe worsening angina Caution within 6 wk of myocardial infarction	Unpleasant taste of unflavored gum Mild sense of buccal mucosal irritation from nicotine absorption when "parked" Hiccups and cough can occur from incorrect use of the gum	Use 4 mg ≥10 cigs/24 h[d] Use 2 mg <10 cigs/24 h[d] Each 4 mg piece = 2 mg absorbed = 2 cigs Each 2 mg piece = 1 mg absorbed = 1 cig 20 cigs = 10 pc 4 mg gum = 20 pc 2 mg gum Take evenly spaced throughout the day to replace need for nicotine Take additional as needed	Tapering may occur naturally as need for nicotine decreases Alternatively, decrease by 1 piece per day every few days	DO NOT CHEW LIKE ORDINARY GUM Recommended use time 20–30 min per piece Alternate chewing and "parking" between cheek and gum (chew until mouth tingles, then "park" for 1 min)

Product	Indications	Precautions	Adverse effects	Dosage	Tapering	Instructions
		Discontinue if tachycardia or palpitations occur	If chewed or swallowed, indigestion and heartburn can occur			Do not eat or drink 15 min before or while using these products Do not smoke while using these products
Nicotine lozenge Commit 4 mg, 2 mg	For patients who smoke less than 1 pack per day acceptable as solo therapy As an adjunctive medication in combination therapy (with nicotine patch or Zyban)	Patients with dry mouth or sicca syndrome may not be able to produce enough saliva to dissolve lozenge Serious arrhythmias or severe worsening angina Caution within 6 wk of myocardial infarction Discontinue if tachycardia or palpitations occur	Mild sense of buccal mucosal irritation from nicotine absorption Hiccups and cough can occur from incorrect use of the lozenge If chewed or swallowed, indigestion and heartburn can occur	Use 4 mg ≥10 cigs/24 h Use 2 mg <10 cigs/24 h Each 4 mg lozenge = 2 mg absorbed = 2 cigs Each 2 mg lozenge = 1 mg absorbed = 1 cig 20 cigs = 10 4 mg lozenges = 20 2 mg lozenges Take evenly spaced throughout the day to replace need for nicotine Take additional as needed	Tapering may occur naturally as need for nicotine decrease. Alternatively, decrease by 1 lozenge per day every few days	DO NOT BITE, CHEW, OR SWALLOW Allow to dissolve in mouth slowly while moving lozenge from side to side Each lozenge takes 20–30 min to dissolve Do not eat or drink 15 min before or while using this product Do not smoke while using this product
Nicotine inhaler Nicotrol Inhaler	For patients who desire the hand-to-mouth feel of a cigarette As an adjunctive medication in combination therapy	Hypersensitivity to menthol Serious arrhythmias or severe worsening angina Caution within 6 wk of myocardial infarction	Mouth and throat irritation; cough	1 cartridge delivers 80 puffs = 2 mg absorbed = 2 cigs 10 cartridges/24 h = 1 pack/d Initial treatment is 6–16 cartridges per day for up to 12 wk	After initial treatment period of 12 wk, gradually reduce dose over the next 6–12 wk	Instruct patient to take 40 puffs, take an hour break, then another 40 puffs per cartridge (manufacturer recommends

(continued on next page)

Table 2
(continued)

Product	Best For	Precautions	Adverse Effects	Dosage	Tapering Schedule	Patient Education
	treatment (with nicotine patch or Zyban)	Discontinue if tachycardia or palpitations occur		Use evenly spread throughout day to replace nicotine requirements		80–100 puffs for 20 min for optimal results, but many patients find such use unpleasant or impractical) Do not use more than 16 cartridges each day Patient is not to puff the inhaler like a cigarette: rather instruct to hold the puff in the mouth for a moment, then to resume regular breathing. This is more akin to cigar or pipe smoking Absorption is via the buccal mucosa, and inappropriate use including attempted inhalation may cause mouth and throat

					irritation and coughing Avoid food and acidic drinks such as coffee, tea, citrus juices, and sodas before and during use Decreased nicotine delivery in cold winter air Do not smoke while using these products
Nicotine nasal spray Nicotrol NS	For patient who needs fast relief or an easy to adjust dose As an adjunctive medication in combination therapy treatment (with nicotine patch or Zyban)	Not recommended in patients with chronic nasal inflammation and obstruction Severe reactive airway disease Serious arrhythmias or severe worsening angina Caution within 6 wk of myocardial infarction Discontinue if tachycardia or palpitations occur	Nasal irritation Sneezing Cough Teary eyes	40 doses = 1 pack/d 1 dose = 1 spray in each nostril = 1 mg of nicotine absorbed Starting dose is 1 or 2 doses per hour, which may be increased up to 40 doses/d	Initial therapy is 3 mo, before tapering for 3–6 mo. Skip doses to taper	Instruct patient to tilt head back and spray Troubling adverse effect of nasal irritation decreases with use Do not smoke while using these products

(continued on next page)

Table 2
(continued)

Product	Best For	Precautions	Adverse Effects	Dosage	Tapering Schedule	Patient Education
Sustained-release bupropion Zyban or Wellbutrin SR Can be used with nicotine replacement therapy	Patients who have difficulty discontinuing cigarette use during quit attempt	Seizure history Current use of Wellbutrin or monoamine oxidase inhibitor Eating disorder (bulimia/anorexia) Alcohol dependence Head trauma Co-use with drugs sharing the cytochrome P450 2B6[e] pathway may be contraindicated Serious arrhythmias or severe worsening angina Caution within 6 wk of myocardial infarction Discontinue if tachycardia or palpitations occur	Insomnia Dry mouth Anxiety Seizures	Start 1–2 wk before quit date. 150 mg/24 h for 3 days then 150 mg twice a day with doses at least 8 h apart For elderly patients, or in cases of polypharmacy 150 mg every morning may be recommended (fewer adverse effects)	No tapering required Usual length of treatment is 7–12 wk	Take second pill in early evening to reduce insomnia Never double dose if a pill is missed Swallow tablet whole; do not crush, divide, or chew Patients should report changes in mood and behavior

[a] Patches are available under various brand names such as Nicoderm CQ and Habitrol, and under generic formulations.

[b] Nicotrol is available in 15-, 10-, and 5-mg doses, and is worn for 16-hour time periods (daytime hours only).

[c] Gum is available under various brand names such as Nicorette, and under generic formulations.

[d] Manufacturer's insert recommends 4 mg ≥25 cigs/24 h, and 2 mg <25 cigs/24 h.

[e] These include most antidepressants (selective serotonin reuptake inhibitors, many tricyclics), β-blockers, antiarrhythmics, and antipsychotics.

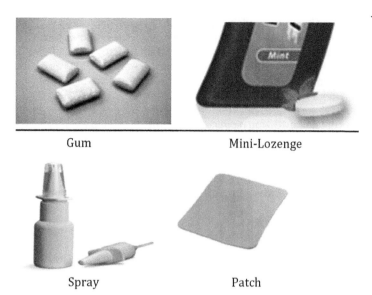

Gum	Mini-Lozenge
Spray	Patch

Fig. 9. Nicotine replacement therapy products.

gastrointestinal tract. Patients with dry mouth or sicca syndrome may not be able to produce enough saliva to dissolve the lozenge. The lozenge is available in regular size (about the size of a US 25-cent coin, or in a mini configuration). The concentrations are the same as for nicotine gum, and lozenges are available in 2-mg and 4-mg sizes.

The lozenge is placed in the mouth and allowed to slowly dissolve while moving it from side to side without chewing. In the first few days of use a mild buccal mucosal irritation can develop.

Dosage for nicotine lozenges:

1. Use 1 lozenge every 1 to 2 hours for the first 6 weeks or until the patient is comfortable with quit attempt
2. Use 1 lozenge every 2 to 4 hours for the next 3 weeks
3. Use 1 lozenge of gum every 4 to 8 hours for the next 3 weeks, until the patient gradually stops usage

If the patient chews on the lozenge and does not allow it to dissolve slowly, the nicotine will be released directly into the saliva, swallowed, and absorbed through the gastrointestinal tract, resulting in severe nausea and tachycardia. Advise your patient not to eat or drink for 15 minutes before or while using the lozenge because this can reduce the absorption of the nicotine. Have your patients contact you or their physician if they develop symptoms of too much nicotine in the body: cold sweats, fainting, confusion, or pounding heart. Occasionally the lozenge may cause mild mucosal irritation. For comprehensive contraindications and adverse effects, refer to individual product inserts and to the Physician's Desk Reference.

Nicotine spray Nicotine nasal spray is aerosolized nicotine contained in a spray pump. The nicotine is delivered to the user by spraying it into the nostrils, and is rapidly absorbed by the nasal membranes inside the nose. The spray device is similar to the type used for over-the-counter decongestant sprays. Because it is rapidly absorbed, the nasal spray delivers the nicotine "hit" much more quickly than other NRTs. This feature makes it attractive to some highly dependent smokers. Do not use for patients with severe reactive airway disease because of the potential to exacerbate bronchospasm.

The nasal spray may not be the most appropriate form of treatment for heavily addicted smokers. For these patients the nasal spray may be helpful as a supplemental source of nicotine when used in combination with another form of NRT or when used in conjunction with a non-nicotine replacement therapy.

Nicotine nasal spray is available by prescription only. It is dispensed in a 10-mL spray bottle containing 100 mg nicotine (10 mg/mL) in an inactive vehicle. Each bottle contains 100 doses.

Dosage for nicotine nasal spray:

1. 1 to 2 doses per hour for 8 weeks. Maximum of 5 doses per hour, or 40 doses (80 sprays) per day for heavily addicted smokers who smoke a pack or more of cigarettes a day
2. Initial therapy is for 3 months
3. Taper for 3 to 6 months; skip doses to taper

To use the nasal spray correctly the patient should blow the nose if it is not clear, tilt the head back slightly and then insert the tip of the bottle into the nostril as far as is comfortable while breathing through the mouth, and then spray once in each nostril; do not sniff or inhale while spraying. If the nose runs, the patient should gently sniff to keep the nasal spray in the nose. The user should wait 2 or 3 minutes before blowing the nose.

Side effects of the spray are usually short lived or are tolerated after the first week. The side effects include irritation of the nose and throat, teary eyes, sneezing, and coughing. For comprehensive contraindications and adverse effects, refer to individual product inserts and to the Physician's Desk Reference.

Nicotine patch The nicotine patch is a patch attached to the skin that uses a membrane to control the rate at which the drug contained in the reservoir within the patch can pass through the skin and into the bloodstream. The nicotine patch works by slowly releasing a constant amount of nicotine into the body through the skin and into the blood while the patch is worn.

The patch is most commonly available in the following concentrations: 21 mg (patients who smoke 10 or more cigarettes a day), 14 mg (patients who smoke less than 10 cigarettes a day), and 7 mg (for tapering only). Dosage scheduling for the nicotine patch is as follows.

It is recommended that one patch be worn for 16 to 24 hours. If your patient craves cigarettes when they wake up in the morning, they should wear the patch for 24 hours. Otherwise, it is acceptable to take it off at bedtime and apply a fresh patch first thing in the morning. In addition, if your patient is having vivid dreams or other sleep disturbances, you may recommend they remove the patch at bedtime and apply a new patch the following morning.

The patch should be applied at approximately the same time each day.

Even if the urge to smoke is gone before the end of the prescribed regimen, completing the full step-down program is important. The step-down treatment period allows a gradual reduction in the amount of nicotine the patient is receiving, rather than a sudden stop, and will increase the chances of quitting successfully.

For the 21-mg patch taper as follows:

Use the 21-mg patch for 6 weeks
Step down to the next size patch, 14 mg, for 2 weeks
Follow by 2 weeks of 7-mg patch

For the 14-mg patch taper as follows:

Use the 14-mg patch for 6 weeks
Step down to the 7-mg patch for 2 weeks

The most common side effects while wearing the patch are skin irritation or discoloration, and vivid dreams or other sleep disturbances. Smoking while using NRTs is not recommended because there is a risk of absorbing too much nicotine and experiencing an overdose. Patients should call your office or their physician if they develop symptoms of nicotine overdose: cold sweats, fainting, confusion, or pounding heart. For comprehensive contraindications and adverse effects, refer to individual product inserts and to the Physician's Desk Reference.

Non-nicotine replacement therapy
Bupropion and varenicline (**Fig. 10**) are therapies that use alternative non-nicotine replacement mechanisms to aid the patient in quitting. In the dental office these medications should be used for patients who have previously tried and failed in a quit attempt when using an NRT, or for patients whose smoking habits place them in a more strongly addicted category.

Bupropion Initially developed and marketed as an antidepressant (Wellbutrin and Wellbutrin SR), Zyban (bupropion hydrochloride) is a sustained-release non-nicotine tablet that aids smoking cessation. It is available as brand name and generic. Although exactly how bupropion works in smoking cessation is not understood, it is known that this prescription-strength medicine alters the brain's chemistry by affecting 2 chemicals in the brain that are believed to help regulate mood, namely dopamine and norepinephrine.[29] Taking bupropion results in diminished nicotine cravings, and often smokers find it easier to quit because smoking loses its appeal. Bupropion should not be used for patients who: (1) are taking other medicines that contain bupropion HCl, (2) have a seizure history or a history of head trauma, (3) have eating disorder(s), or (4) are taking a monoamine oxidase inhibitors. It is important that you ask about all

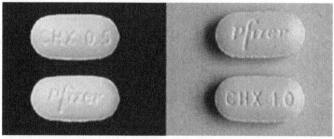

Varenicline (Chantix)

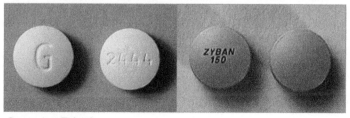

Bupropion (Zyban)

Fig. 10. Alternative non-nicotine replacement therapy.

medications, prescription or over-the-counter, that your patients are taking or plan to take while taking bupropion. Bupropion should not be used by patients who are taking medications that are metabolized by the cytochrome P450 2B6 pathway. It is important not to take medicines that may increase the risk of seizure.[29]

The risks of using bupropion for smoking cessation should be weighed against the benefits. Bupropion is effective in helping patients to quit smoking. The benefits of quitting smoking are substantive. The Food and Drug Administration (FDA) requires the following warning to be provided for bupropion prescriptions[30]:

> *Advise patients and caregivers that the patient using bupropion for smoking cessation should contact a healthcare provider immediately if agitation, depressed mood, or changes in behavior or thinking that are not typical for the patient are observed, or if the patient develops suicidal ideation or suicidal behavior. In many post-marketing cases, resolution of symptoms after discontinuation of bupropion was reported, although in some cases the symptoms persisted, therefore, ongoing monitoring and supportive care should be provided until symptoms resolve.*

Dosage for bupropion:

1. Start 1 to 2 weeks before quit date
2. First 3 days 150 mg/24 h
3. After first 3 days 0.5 mg twice per day (once in the morning and once in the evening)
4. After first 7 days 150 mg twice per day with doses at least 8 hours apart

Although it is not considered dangerous to smoke and use bupropion at the same time, continuing to smoke after the quit date will seriously reduce the chances of success.

Varenicline Varenicline is a non-nicotine prescription tablet designed to help adults stop smoking. Varenicline is the generic name for Chantix. Varenicline works through mimicking nicotine by stimulating nicotine receptors to release dopamine while at the same time blocking nicotine from stimulating the nicotine receptors. Although the varenicline dopamine release is modulated and less than what a smoker would receive from having a cigarette, it is longer lasting and remains throughout the day as long as it is taken as directed. Varenicline should not be used with: (1) breastfeeding women, (2) persons with severe renal impairment, or (3) in individuals with prior or current psychiatric illness.[31]

The risks of using varenicline for smoking cessation should be weighed against the benefits. Varenicline is effective in helping patients to quit smoking. The benefits of quitting smoking are substantive. The FDA requires the following warning to be provided for varenicline prescriptions[30]:

> *Advise patients and caregivers that the patient using varenicline for smoking cessation should contact a healthcare provider immediately if agitation, depressed mood, or changes in behavior or thinking that are not typical for the patient are observed, or if the patient develops suicidal ideation or suicidal behavior. In many post-marketing cases, resolution of symptoms after discontinuation of varenicline was reported, although in some cases the symptoms persisted, therefore, ongoing monitoring and supportive care should be provided until symptoms resolve.*

Dosage of varenicline:

1. Start 1 week before quit date
2. First 3 days 0.5 mg/24 h

3. Next 4 day 0.5 mg twice per day (once in the morning and once in the evening)
4. After first 7 days 1 mg twice per day (once in the morning and once in the evening)

Varenicline should be taken on a full stomach and with a full glass (8 ounces) of water. One dose should be taken in the morning and one dose in the evening.

Patients should be treated for 12 weeks. An additional 12-week course is recommended for successful patients to increase the likelihood of long-term abstinence.

If, for the aforementioned reasons, varenicline must be discontinued, this does not mean that tobacco-cessation counseling should cease. If at first you don't succeed, try, try again. A failed quit attempt is not a treatment failure. It can take multiple attempts for the patient to successfully quit. Instead of giving up hope, you should introduce a different treatment regimen, such as combination NRT, and encourage the patient to tackle tobacco use with this new approach.

Combination therapy

Combination therapy should be considered for patients who have failed prior pharmacotherapeutic-assisted tobacco-cessation attempts or for heavy smokers (more than 1 pack of cigarettes a day).[32] Current product information does not support the use of more than one NRT; however, there is pharmacologic rationale to support the use of multiple NRT regimens. NRT regimens typically provide a lower plasma level of nicotine than a patient would receive from cigarette smoking. Many patients fail in a quit attempt, particularly in the first few weeks, because their nicotine levels are too low and they cannot overcome their craving for nicotine.

There are 2 approaches to combination therapy: NRT based or bupropion plus a short-acting NRT.

NRT-based combination therapy should include: (1) a long-acting source of nicotine such as a nicotine patch and (2) a short-acting treatment such as nicotine gum, lozenge, inhaler, or spray.

Bupropion plus a short-acting NRTs should include bupropion (Zyban) combined with any of the short-acting NRTs (nicotine gum, lozenge, inhaler, spray).

Arrange

For those patients who make a commitment to quit, a call from the office on or before the patient's quit date has proved to be a key factor in patients successfully quitting. For those who are not quite ready to quit, it is essential to discuss their tobacco use at every visit; each time it is discussed, the patient may move closer to making a decision to quit.

Quit lines are also available to patients. Quit lines are toll-free help lines whereby a patient can talk to a counselor about ways to stop or arrange to have information on how to quit mailed to their home. Quit lines also can link the patient to local services for help as needed.

Many quit lines can provide information for special groups, such as:

Pregnant women
Users of smokeless (chew and snuff) tobacco
People who want to help a friend or family member quit
Different racial or ethnic groups
Teen smokers

Anyone in the United States can call 1-800-QUIT-NOW (1-800-784-8669). Many states also have their own quit lines. If your state has one, your patient will be automatically redirected to it when he or she calls 1-800-QUIT-NOW.

The US Government has a Web site, http://www.smokefree.gov, dedicated to helping people give up tobacco. It links to the North American quit line site, which includes an interactive map (http://www.naquitline.org/index.asp?dbsection=map&dbid=1). Just click on your state. Your patient will get information on quit line phone numbers, hours of operation, eligibility requirements for counseling and free medications, types of counseling provided, and languages spoken. Most states can use translators to provide counseling in more than 140 languages.

Another way to help patients is to give them self-help written materials to take home. Take the time to look at the patient materials before distributing them. Some patients may ask you what information is contained in the brochures.

Information on ordering self-help materials for patients can be obtained by contacting any of the following:

The Agency for Healthcare Research and Quality (AHRQ), 800-358-9295. http://www.ahrq.gov/

The American Cancer Society, 800-227-2345. http://www.cancer.org

The Centers for Disease Control and Prevention (CDC), 800-CDC-1311. http://www.cdc.gov

The National Cancer Institute (NCI), 800-4-CANCER. http://www.cancer.gov

Web site created by the Tobacco Control Research Branch of the National Cancer Institute, with contributions from other agencies and organizations such as the CDC, the American Cancer Society, and NCI. www.smokefree.gov

BARRIERS TO CESSATION ACTIVITIES

While it is widely accepted among dental professionals that tobacco use has a direct impact on the oral cavity and overall health, the profession has been slow to adopt the US Public Health Service recommendations that were published in 2000.[5] Dental clinicians often cite patient resistance, time constraints, effectiveness of tobacco-cessation interventions, access to educational materials, and reimbursement as barriers to incorporating tobacco cessation into dental practice.

Public health agencies and professional dental organizations including the American Dental Association (ADA) have sought to reduce these perceived barriers and increase adoption by dental clinicians of the 5 A's into routine clinical practice. Formal tobacco-cessation training offered to clinicians has been found to increase provider knowledge and self-efficacy. In addition, training that involves showing clinicians how to use brief interventions in an efficient manner have been reported to reduce concerns about lack of time.[33] Educational materials on tobacco cessation that have been made available by federal and state agencies have helped to address some of the concerns expressed by clinicians about lack of materials. Patient resistance to tobacco-cessation interventions has not been found to be an issue; on the contrary, surveys of dental patients show that they feel that their clinicians should talk to them about the effects of smoking and that they would welcome advice about quitting. Tobacco-cessation counseling by dental clinicians has a dental treatment code assigned to it by the ADA, CDT code D1320, "tobacco counseling for the control and prevention of oral disease." Unfortunately, major dental insurers presently do not reimburse for this treatment code. As the dental profession continues to embrace tobacco cessation as an essential service that improves oral and systemic health, coverage for this intervention will inevitably become a component of dental insurance plans.

SUMMARY

Tobacco has a profound impact on the oral cavity. It is directly related to many oral conditions, lesions, and neoplastic activity. The dental provider is in the unique position to provide advice on quitting and showing the patient the oral effects of smoking. The dental clinician sees the typical patient for multiple visits, enabling reinforcement and encouragement with the attempt to quit. Finally, the dentist who assists by prescribing a pharmacotherapeutic agent has been shown to increase successful quit attempts by as much as 2 to 3 times. The ultimate goal is an improvement in oral and systemic health, an objective that the dental team can achieve in the context of a regular office visit.

REFERENCES

1. Doll R, Peto R, Boreham J, et al. Mortality in relation to smoking: 50 years' observations on male British doctors. BMJ 2004;328:1519. http://dx.doi.org/10.1136/bmj.38142.554479.AE.
2. Centers for Disease Control and Prevention. Annual smoking attributable mortality, years of potential life lost, and productivity losses—United States, 1997-2001. MMWR Morb Mortal Wkly Rep 2005;24(5):477–87.
3. Centers for Disease Control and Prevention. Cigarette smoking among adults—United States, 2000. MMWR Morb Mortal Wkly Rep 2002;51(29):642–5.
4. Hammond D, McDonald PW, Fong GT, et al. Do smokers know how to quit? Knowledge and perceived effectiveness of cessation assistance as predictors of cessation behavior. Addiction 2004;99(8):1042–8.
5. Fiore MC, Jaen CR, Baker TB, et al. Treating tobacco use and dependence: clinical practice guideline. Rockville (MD): U.S. Department of Health and Human Services, Public Health Service; 2008.
6. Mucci LA, Brooks DR. Lower use of dental services among long term cigarette smokers. J Epidemiol Community Health 2001;55(6):389–93.
7. Rea DR, Heckbert SR, Kaplan RC, et al. Smoking status and risk for recurrent coronary events after myocardial infarction. Ann Intern Med 2002;137:494–500.
8. U.S. Department of Health and Human Services. The health consequences of involuntary exposure to tobacco smoke: a report of the Surgeon General. U.S. Department of Health and Human Services, Centers for Disease Control and Prevention, Coordinating Center for Health Promotion, National Center for Chronic Disease Prevention and Health Promotion, Office on Smoking and Health. Atlanta: Georgia; 2006.
9. Alberg AJ, Ford JG, Samet JM. Epidemiology of lung cancer: ACCP evidence-based clinical practice guidelines (2nd edition). Chest 2007;132(Suppl 3):29S–55S.
10. Centers for Disease Control and Prevention (CDC). Vital signs: nonsmokers' exposure to secondhand smoke—United States, 1999-2008. MMWR Morb Mortal Wkly Rep 2010;59(35):1141–6.
11. O'Connor RJ. Non-cigarette tobacco products: what have we learnt and where are we headed? Tob Control 2012;21(2):181–90.
12. Nelson DE, Mowery P, Tomar S, et al. Trends in smokeless tobacco use among adults and adolescents in the United States. Am J Public Health 2006;96(5):897.
13. Papapanou PN. Periodontal diseases: epidemiology. Ann Periodontol 1996;1:1–36.
14. McNeill A, Bedl R, Islam S, et al. Levels of toxins in oral tobacco products in the UK. Tob Control 2006;15(1):64–7.
15. Bergström J, Eliasson S, Dock J. A 10-year prospective study of tobacco smoking and periodontal health. J Periodontol 2000;71:1338–47.
16. Ah MK, Johnson GK, Kaldahl WB, et al. The effect of smoking on the response to periodontal therapy. J Clin Periodontol 1994;21:91–7.

17. Preber H, Bergström J. Effect of cigarette smoking on periodontal healing following surgical therapy. J Clin Periodontol 1990;17:324–8.

18. Tonetti MS, Pini PG, Cortellini P. Effect of cigarette smoking on periodontal healing following GTR in infrabony defects. A preliminary retrospective study. J Clin Periodontol 1995;22:229–34.

19. Bolin A, Eklund G, Frithiof L, et al. The effect of changed smoking habits on marginal alveolar bone loss. A longitudinal study. Swed Dent J 1993;17:211–6.

20. Tomar SL, Asma S. Smoking-attributable periodontitis in the United States: findings from NHANES III. National Health and Nutrition Examination Survey. J Periodontol 2000;71:743–51.

21. Tomar SL, Winn DM. Chewing tobacco use and dental caries among U.S. men. J Am Dent Assoc 1999;30(11):1601–10.

22. Taybos G. Oral changes associated with tobacco use. Am J Med Sci 2003; 326(4):179–82.

23. Wingo PA, Tong T, Bolden S. Cancer statistics. CA Cancer J Clin 1995;45:8–30.

24. Ries, LAG, Miler, BA, Hankey, BF, et al, editors. SEER cancer statistics review, 1973–91: tables and graphs. Bethesda: National Cancer Institute (NIH Publication no. 94-2789), 1994.

25. Centers for Disease Control and Prevention. Cigarette smoking—attributable mortality and years of potential life lost-United States. 1990. MMWR Morb Mortal Wkly Rep 1993;42:645–9.

26. Neville BW, Day TA. Oral cancer and precancerous lesions. CA Cancer J Clin 2002;52:195–215.

27. Greer RO. Oral manifestations of smokeless tobacco use. Otolaryngol Clin North Am 2011;44(1):31–56, v.

28. Hedin CA. Smokers' melanosis. Occurrence and localization in the attached gingiva. Arch Dermatol 1977;113(11):1533–8.

29. Hughes JR, Stead LF, Lancaster T. Antidepressants for smoking cessation. Cochrane Database Syst Rev 2007;1:CD000031.

30. Available at: http://www.fda.gov/Drugs/DrugSafety/PostmarketDrugSafety InformationforPatientsandProviders/DrugSafetyInformationforHeathcareProfessionals/ ucm169986.htm. Accessed May 7, 2012.

31. Cahill K, Stead LF, Lancaster T. Nicotine receptor partial agonists for smoking cessation. Cochrane Database Syst Rev 2011;(2):CD006103.

32. Cofta-Woerpel L, Wright KL, Wetter DW. Smoking cessation 3: multicomponent interventions. Behav Med 2007;32(4):135–49.

33. Patel AM, Blanchard SB, Christen AG, et al. A survey of U.S. periodontists' knowledge, attitudes, and behaviors related to tobacco cessation interventions. J Periodontol 2011;82:367–76.

Dermatology of the Head and Neck: Skin Cancer and Benign Skin Lesions

Monica Halem, MD[a],*, Chanté Karimkhani, BA, BA[b]

KEYWORDS

- Skin cancer • Benign skin lesions • Diagnosis

KEY POINTS

- By becoming aware of common lesions and their phenotypic presentation, dental professionals are empowered to detect suspicious dermatologic lesions in unaware patients.
- Skin lesions are extremely common, and early detection of dangerous lesions makes skin cancer one of the most highly curable malignancies.
- Dentists can have an impact on the health of their patients by examining the skin, making the appropriate referral, and following up with the patient to determine if they have seen a dermatologist.

INTRODUCTION TO THE SKIN

The skin is the largest organ in the body, comprising 18% of body weight and covering a surface area of 1.8 m^2, and fulfills many vital roles for the human body.[1] It provides protection from the external world, including protection from physical insults, microorganisms, and ultraviolet (UV) irradiation. The skin also fosters a homeostatic internal body environment, ranging from fluid balance to thermoregulation, vitamin D production, and immune regulation. The skin is composed of 3 primary layers: the epidermis, the dermis, and the subcutaneous fat (**Fig. 1**). The epidermis is a stratified squamous epithelium derived from ectoderm and is composed of 4 principle cell types: keratinocytes, melanocytes, Langerhans cells, and Merkel cells. Skin cancers arise when proliferation involving these cell types becomes dysregulated. The epidermis is separated from the dermis by a basement membrane. The dermis provides structural support and nutrients via connective tissue, rich vascularization, and innervation. The underlying subcutaneous fat is a meshwork of loose connective tissue and fat that provides insulation for the internal body systems and energy storage. The

[a] Department of Dermatology, Columbia University, 161 Fort Washington Avenue, 12th Floor, New York, NY 10032, USA; [b] Columbia University College of Physicians and Surgeons, 630 West 168th St, New York, NY 10032, USA
* Corresponding author.
E-mail address: mlh2166@columbia.edu

Dent Clin N Am 56 (2012) 771–790
http://dx.doi.org/10.1016/j.cden.2012.07.005
0011-8532/12/$ – see front matter © 2012 Published by Elsevier Inc.

dental.theclinics.com

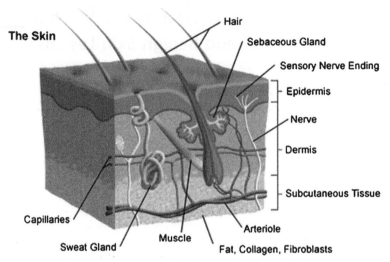

Fig. 1. The skin has 3 layers: the epidermis, the dermis, and the subcutaneous fat. (*From* Zhang A, Obagi S. Complications in Cosmetic Facial Surgery Diagnosis and Management of Skin Resurfacing–Related Complications. Oral and Maxillofacial Surgery Clinics 2009; 21(1):1–12.)

subcutis and the dermis also contain important structures such as sebaceous glands, hair follicles, eccrine glands, and apocrine glands. This basic introduction to skin histology provides a foundation for an understanding of skin pathology ranging from skin cancer and precursor lesions to benign skin proliferations.

NONMELANOMA SKIN CANCER

Skin cancer is broadly categorized into 2 main subtypes: Nonmelanoma skin cancer (NMSC), and malignant melanoma. NMSC consists of basal cell carcinomas (BSCs) and squamous cell carcinomas (SCCs). Trends indicate that the incidence of NMSC is rapidly increasing worldwide, affecting more than one million Americans per year.[2] More than 3.5 million skin cancers are diagnosed annually.[3] The estimated average lifetime risk for Caucasians to develop NMSC is upwards of 30%.[4] BSC and SCC are the 2 most common forms of skin cancer, but both are easily treated if detected early. A recent study found that BSC and SCC are increasing in men and women younger than 40 years of age. In the study, BSC increased faster in young women than in young men.[5] In humans, there are more skin cancers than all other cancers, and current estimates are that 1 in 5 Americans will develop skin cancer in their lifetime.[6] Once an individual has developed one NMSC, they are more likely to develop another. One meta-analysis estimates that these patients have a 44% risk of developing an additional skin cancer within 3 years.[7]

Risk Factors

There are several risk factors for developing NMSC (**Box 1**).[8] NMSC has a predilection for patients with (1) a history of intense UV radiation exposure during childhood (0–19 years of age), (2) Fitzpatrick skin types I–II, (3) blonde or red hair color, (4) light eye color, and (5) chronic photodamaged skin, especially in the head and neck region.[9] The most significant risk factor for the development of NMSC appears to be exposure to UV radiation. However, the timing, pattern, and amount of exposure to UV radiation also seem to be important. The risk of disease is significantly increased by exposure to

| **Box 1** |
| **Risk factors for development of NMSC** |
| *Risk Factors for NMSC* |
| Ultraviolet radiation |
| Arsenic exposure |
| Ionizing radiation |
| Tanning bed use |
| Red or blond hair |
| Light eye color |
| Fitzpatrick skin types I–II |
| Immunosuppression |
| Genodermatoses |
| Decreasing latitude |

UV radiation during childhood and adolescence[10] as well as intense intermittent and chronic cumulative sun exposure.[11] Physical factors, including fair complexion, hair and eye color, influence responsiveness to UV radiation and also act as independent risk factors.[12] Other risk factors include a history of diagnostic or therapeutic radiation,[13] arsenic exposure,[14] immunosuppressive therapy for organ transplant recipients,[15] psoralen and UVA radiation,[16] exposure to human papilloma virus, and various genodermatoses such as Gorlin syndrome and xeroderma pigmentosum (see **Box 1**).[17] It has been estimated that 16% of renal transplant patients will develop NMSC, SCC more than BCC, and the risk increases with the length of their immunosuppression.[18] The incidence of BCC in organ transplant recipients is 5 to 10 times greater than its incidence in the general population, whereas the incidence of SCC is 65 to 250 times greater.[19] In the next few sections the authors discuss in detail the 2 types of NMSC, BSC and SCC.

BASAL CELL CARCINOMA

Cutaneous BCC is the most ubiquitous cancer affecting humans worldwide.[20] Over 1 million cases were detected in the United States in 2010, 95% between ages 40 and 79.[21] BCC accounts for approximately 60% to 75% of all skin cancers.[22] BCC is an indolent, locally invasive, malignant epithelial neoplasm arising from the basilar layer of the epidermis.[23] It slowly progresses, with projections of microtumor spreading in a three-dimensional manner throughout the papillary and reticular dermis,[24] and rarely leads to metastasis. One reason for the apparent limitation to the dermal layer of skin may be tumor dependence on the stromal environment of the dermal fibroblast. BCC is thought to be composed of aberrant follicular germinative cells, also known as trichoblasts, because of its morphologic and immunohistochemical similarities to hair follicle structures.[25]

Pathogenesis

The pathogenesis of BCC is related to genetic mutation. The most common mutated genes in BCC pathogenesis include the PTCH gene on chromosome 9q and point mutations in p53 on chromosome 17p.[26] Both PTCH and p53 are tumor suppressor genes that encode proteins responsible for preventing cell cycle progression. The role that the PTCH gene plays in BCC pathogenesis is highlighted by nevoid BCC syndrome, which results from an inherited autosomal dominant mutation in PTCH gene. People affected by this disorder classically develop hundreds of BCCs, including palmar and plantar pits, odontogenic keratocysts of the jaws, skeletal abnormalities, and calcification of the falx cerebri.

Clinical Presentation

BCC characteristically arises in body areas exposed to the sun and is most common on the head and neck, followed by the trunk, arms, and legs. In addition, BCCs have been reported in unusual sites, including the axillae, breasts, perianal area, genitalia, palms, and soles. BCCs have been classified into 4 main types according to clinical and histopathologic features: superficial, nodular, micronodular, and infiltrative or morpheaform (**Table 1**). In a retrospective study of more than 10,000 cases of diagnosed BCCs, 79% were nodular, 15% were superficial, and 6% were morpheaform.[27] The nodular and morpheaform types were observed on the head and neck 90% to 95% of the time, whereas 46% of superficial BCCs occurred on the trunk. Nodular BCC is the classic form, which most often presents as a pearly pink to white dome-shaped papule surrounded by a well-demarcated rolled border; prominent telangiectatic vessels may superficially traverse the lesion usually present on the face and ears (**Fig. 2**). Patients often describe this papule as a nonhealing "pimple" that bleeds occasionally. Superficial BCC presents as a scaly erythematous patch or plaque usually on the trunk or extremities (**Fig. 3**). The morpheaform type, also known as sclerosing, fibrosing, or infiltrative BCC, typically appears as an indurated, whitish, scarlike plaque with indistinct margins (**Fig. 4**). This type of BCC is slightly tougher to diagnose because of its ill-defined margins and often present later. The value of classifying the histologic appearance of BCC lies in the relationship between histologic subtype and clinical behavior. Aggressive histologic variants include micronodular, infiltrative, basosquamous, morpheaform, and mixed subtypes.[28] Nodular and superficial subtypes generally have a less aggressive clinical course.

Recurrence and Metastasis Factors

The greatest risk of BCC recurrence has been shown to be within the first 5 years after treatment.[29] Risk factors for recurrence include a tumor diameter greater than 2 cm,

Table 1 Types of BCC	
BCC Varieties	**Unique Features**
Nodular	Most common BCC (60%), raised and translucent papule or nodule with telangiectasias, often on face, may ulcerate, may be pigmented (hard to tell from melanoma)
Superficial	Erythematous macule or thin plaque, trunk and extremities>head and neck
Morpheaform	Looks like scleroderma
Cystic	Clear or blue-gray, exude clear fluid if punctured
Basosquamous	Behave more like SCC (more aggressive and destructive), increased metastases
Micronodular	Infiltrate dermis
Fibroepithelioma of Pinkus	Pink plaque on lower back, looks like amelanotic melanoma

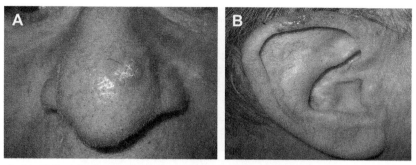

Fig. 2. (*A, B*) Nodular basal cell carcinoma: pearly pink to white dome-shaped papule.

location on the central part of the face or ears, long-standing duration, incomplete excision, an aggressive histologic growth pattern, and perineural or perivascular involvement.[30] Tumors with subclinical extension or indistinct borders have a higher recurrence rate than more limited or well-defined tumors. Metastasis of BCC is rare, with metastatic rates ranging from 0.003% to 0.5%.[31] Fewer than 500 cases have been reported in the literature.[32]

SQUAMOUS CELL CARCINOMA

SCC is the second most common skin cancer and represents 20% of all NMSC cases.[33] It is estimated that the lifetime risk for developing an SCC in Caucasian men is 9% to 14% and in women, 4% to 9%.[34] A significant rise in the incidence of SCC over the past 2 decades has been documented.[35] SCCs arise from the epidermis with atypical keratinocyte cells that can invade the dermis and progress to metastasize. Unlike BCC, SCC has a significant risk of metastasis and can be fatal.

Pathogenesis

SCC has a classical precursor lesion, the actinic keratosis (AK). AKs are precancerous lesions defined by histologic atypical keratinocytes that do not encompass the entire epidermis. In contrast, an SCC has full-thickness keratinocyte atypia. AKs are one of the most frequently seen lesions in any dermatology practice. They are more common in lighter-skinned persons with a predilection for areas of increased sun exposure

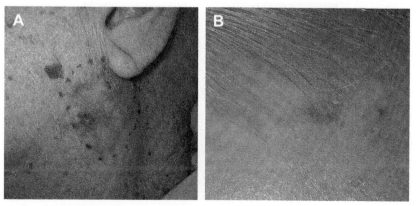

Fig. 3. (*A, B*) Superficial BCC: scaly erythematous plaque.

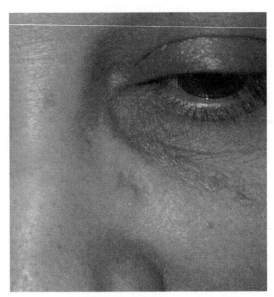

Fig. 4. Morpheaform BCC: indurated scarlike plaque.

including the head, neck, and upper extremities. AK may be identified as rough, erythematous papules with white or yellow scale that are more easily felt than seen (**Fig. 5**). They are usually in the presence of a background of photodamage to the skin. Approximately 2% to 10% of all AKs evolve into invasive SCC.[36] There is a 10% lifetime risk of a person with multiple AKs to develop a SCC.[37] This risk also depends on the number of AK lesions and the length of time they are present. Options for treating AKs include cryosurgery, electrodessication and curettage, and topical chemotherapy. SCC is believed to derive from a single transformed cell of the keratinocyte lineage in the epidermis. Exposure to UV radiation is the most common cause of SCC. Repetitive UV irradiation hitting vulnerable keratinocytes induces mutations in the DNA of the p53 tumor-suppressor gene, leading to tumor formation.[38] Other factors that lead to the formation of SCC are exposure to ionizing radiation, infection with human papilloma virus, exposure to chemical agents such as arsenic, and intake

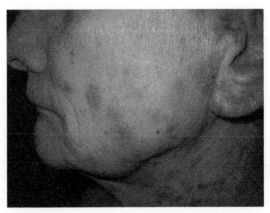

Fig. 5. AK: rough, erythematous papules with white or yellow scale.

of immunosuppressive medications as seen in organ transplant recipients. Organ transplant recipients develop SCC more often than BCC in contrast to the general population.

Clinical Presentation

SCCs are identified as an erythematous, pink, scaling plaque, papule, or nodule on sun-exposed skin that may have ulceration (**Fig. 6**). Lesions can be crusted plaques or firm nodules as well. They most commonly occur on the head and neck, but often occur on the trunk.[39] Patients often describe their lesions as nonhealing wounds that bleed periodically and may or not be painful. SCCs are also more likely to develop in injured skin or in skin that is chronically diseased such as long-standing ulcers, radiation dermatitis, or vaccination scars.[39] These lesions also have a tendency to develop in mucocutaneous sites such as the lip and oral mucosa. SCCs in these areas have increased metastatic potential.

Recurrence and Metastasis Factors

Unlike BCC, SCC is associated with increased metastatic potential and worse prognosis. The 5-year rate of recurrence is 8%, and the 5-year rate of metastasis is 5%.[40] Risk factors for increased recurrence and metastatic potential include large lesions (>2 cm), poorly defined borders, a rapidly growing tumor, poorly differentiated histology, and tumors located on the head and neck but specifically the lip, eyelid, and ear. The presence of immunosuppression and perineural involvement on pathology also increases metastatic risk.[39]

TREATMENT OF NMSC

NMSC is one of the most treatable cancers with an excellent prognosis. However, proper treatment requires the early detection of suspicious lesions and follow-up

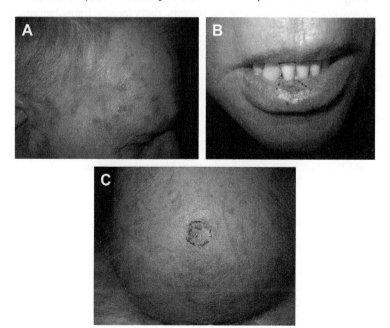

Fig. 6. (A–C) SCC: erythematous pink, scaling plaque, papule, or nodule.

with a dermatologist, plastic surgeon, or other specialist. As with any medical workup, the primary goal of the dermatologic examination is a thorough history-taking and physical examination. Suspicious lesions are biopsied, and the specimen is then sent for pathologic examination, which ideally will yield a diagnosis and allow for stratification of the lesion according to risk. Following diagnosis, numerous techniques are available for treatment, which can be divided into surgical and nonsurgical (**Table 2**). Choice of treatment should take into consideration tumor type, location, histologic growth pattern, and whether the tumor is primary or recurrent. Surgical approaches include curettage and electrodesiccation, cryosurgery, surgical excision, and Mohs micrographic surgery. The most frequently used method for treatment of BCC is surgical excision, which has the advantage of histologic evaluation of the margins of the specimen, although vertical processing allows visualization of less than 1% of the entire specimen margin.[41] Mohs micrographic surgery remains the gold standard because of its highest cure rate, complete histologic analysis of tumor margins using horizontal sectioning techniques, and preservation of normal tissue (**Fig. 7**).[42] Electrodessication and curettage is easy to perform, cost-effective, and cosmetically acceptable; however, cure rates are much less and are highly dependent on technique and experience. Nonsurgical approaches include radiotherapy, topical and injectable therapy, and photodynamic therapy. Radiotherapy is an important option for patients who are not surgical candidates, although its use may be limited because of the risk of side effects. Newer topical therapies such as imiquimod and photodynamic therapy have been shown to be useful for superficial lesions. However, there are few randomized controlled studies comparing different skin cancer treatments, and much of the published literature has low patient numbers and short-term follow-up.[43] Cryosurgery, involving freezing of the lesion with liquid nitrogen, is the mainstay treatment for AKs, the precursor lesion of SCC. Additional nonsurgical treatments include novel topical and intralesional injection therapies using compounds such as 5-fluorouracil. The management of high-risk skin cancers involves a multidisciplinary team of dermatologists, surgical oncologists, medical oncologists, pathologists, transplant physicians, and radiation oncologists.

Proper follow-up and screening are necessary for patients who have had a previous NMSC. The rates of recurrence for BCC and SCC tend to be around 30% to 40% in 5 years after treatment for a primary tumor.[7] These follow-ups require 3- to 6-month skin examinations and education awareness of recurrent disease.

MELANOMA
Incidence

Melanoma is the most dangerous type of skin cancer with an incidence and overall mortality rate that has been rising worldwide. Melanoma incidence rates have been increasing for at least 30 years. In the most recent time period, rapid increases have

Table 2 NMSC treatment options	
Surgical	**Nonsurgical**
Surgical excision	Topical imiquimod
Mohs micrographic surgical excision	Photodynamic therapy
Electrodesiccation and curettage	Radiotherapy
Cryosurgery	Laser therapy

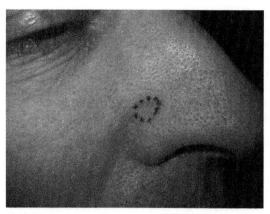

Fig. 7. Outline of a basal cell carcinoma that requires MOHS micrographic surgery.

occurred among young, white women (3% per year since 1992 in those aged between 15 and 39 years) and white adults aged 65 years and older (5.1% per year since 1985 in men and 4.1% per year since 1975 in women).[6,44] This increase is more rapid than for any other malignancy. Melanoma is one of the most common malignancies found in young adults. It is the leading cancer in women aged 25 to 30 years and second only to breast cancer in women aged 30 to 35 years.[45] Overall, one in 59 men and women will be diagnosed with melanoma during their lifetime, one in 39 for Caucasian men and one in 58 for Caucasian women.[46] One American dies of melanoma almost every hour, and approximately 75% of all skin cancer deaths are from melanoma.[6]

Pathogenesis

Melanoma represents abnormal proliferation of pigment-producing melanocytes, which are located primarily in the skin with smaller populations found in the eyes, ears, gastrointestinal tract, leptomeninges, and oral and genital mucus membranes. Current theories regarding melanoma pathogenesis involve the accumulation of progressive genetic mutations that modify cell differentiation, proliferation, and death, ultimately increasing susceptibility to the damaging effects of UV radiation.[47] Although approximately 70% of melanomas develop de novo, 30% arise from melanocytic nevi precursors.[48] Stepwise progression to cellular atypia and pleomorphism represent intermediate steps in the pathway of melanoma development.[49] In particular, mutations in the proto-oncogene BRAF are associated with melanoma development in intermittently sun-exposed skin, whereas c-KIT mutations are associated with melanoma development in chronically sun-exposed or unexposed skin sites.[50] Approximately 25% of rare familial variants of melanoma in fair-skinned people are associated with high-penetrance gene mutations in CDKN2A, involving p53 and Rb molecular pathways.[51] However, genetic testing for these melanoma-susceptible genotypes is not currently advised outside of research protocols.

Risk Factors

Genetic risk factors for melanoma include a family or personal history of melanoma, increased numbers and unusual or changing moles, lightly pigmented skin, tendency to burn or inability to tan, red hair color, and DNA repair defective syndromes such as xeroderma pigmentosa.[48] The development of melanoma is also highly influenced by the environmental risk factors, including intense intermittent sun exposure of unaccustomed skin, sunburn, life in equatorial latitudes, and exposure to UV radiation of any type. Melanoma etiopathogenesis may be more significantly induced by UVA more than UVB radiation, which has significant implications for UVA tanning beds and raises the importance of sunscreens with broad-spectrum coverage of both UVB and UVA.[52] Exposure to tanning beds increases the risk of melanoma, especially in women aged 45 years or younger.[53] People who have more than 50 moles, atypical moles, or a family history of melanoma are at an increased risk of developing melanoma.[21]

Clinical Presentation

Primary cutaneous melanoma is classified into 4 subtypes: superficial spreading, nodular, lentigo maligna, and acral lentiginous (**Table 3**).[1] Superficial spreading melanoma is the most common subtype, comprising 60% to 70% of all diagnosed melanomas (**Fig. 8**). It can arise on any site, but has a predilection for the trunk on men and legs on women. Superficial spreading melanoma is diagnosed most often between age 30 and 50 years. Approximately half of superficial spreading melanomas begin in a preexisting nevus. The lesion progresses to an asymptomatic brown-black macule with color variations and irregular borders and grows in a radial pattern. Nodular melanoma represents 15% to 30% of all melanomas (**Fig. 9**).[54] This variant commonly arises on the trunk, head, or neck and is diagnosed most often in the sixth decade. In contrast to superficial spreading melanoma, nodular melanoma is characterized by rapid vertical growth instead of radial growth. It commonly present as a blue-black (sometimes pink-red) nodule, which may be ulcerated or bleeding, that has undergone rapid vertical growth over the last several months. Lentigo maligna is a less common melanoma subtype, comprising 5% to 15% of all melanomas and

Table 3 Melanoma subtypes		
Melanoma Subtypes	**Unique Features**	**Precursor Lesions**
Superficial spreading	60%–70%, any site (trunk of men and legs of women), radial growth, diagnosed most often between age 30 and 50 years	Begins as asymptomatic brown-black macule with color variations and irregular borders
Nodular	15%–30%, any site (trunk, head, neck), no radial growth, rapid vertical growth, diagnosed most often in sixth decade	Present as blue-black (sometimes pink-red) nodule (may be ulcerated or bleeding) that has grown rapidly over last several months
Lentigo maligna	5%–15%, face (especially nose and cheeks), slow radial growth, diagnosed most often in seventh decade	Occurs on chronically sun-exposed skin, begins as asymmetric and slow-growing brown-black macule with color variations and irregular border, may develop from precursor lesion lentigo maligna (5% progress)
Acral lentiginous	5%–10%, palms/soles/nail unit, radial growth, most common melanoma in darker skin types, diagnosed most often in seventh decade	Presents as asymmetric brown-black macule with color variation and irregular borders, disproportionate percentage of acral lentiginous melanomas diagnosed at advanced stage, nail involvement presents as nail band or even hyperpigmentation in hyponychium

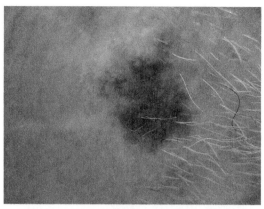

Fig. 8. Superficial spreading melanoma: asymptomatic brown-black macule with color variations and irregular borders.

is found primarily on the face, especially the nose and cheeks. Lentigo maligna undergoes slow radial growth and is diagnosed most often in the seventh decade. It tends to occur on chronically sun-exposed skin, beginning as an asymmetric and slow-growing brown-black macule with color variations and irregular borders. The least common melanoma subtype, acral lentiginous melanoma, comprises 5% to 10% of all melanomas and affects the palms, soles, and nail unit (**Fig. 10**). Acral melanoma is the most common subtype in darker skin types and is diagnosed most often in the seventh decade. It presents as an asymmetric, brown-black macule with color variation, irregular borders, and radial growth. Nail involvement presents as a nail band or hyperpigmentation in the hyponychium. A disproportionate number of acral melanomas are diagnosed at an advanced stage.

TREATMENT OF MELANOMA
Workup

The approach to a patient with suspected melanoma always begins with a thorough medical history, specifically covering potential melanoma risk factors, genetic syndromes for cancer predisposition, and a detailed history of the specific lesion.

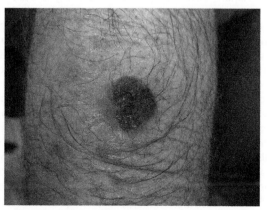

Fig. 9. Nodular melanoma: a blue-black (sometimes pink-red) nodule, which may be ulcerated or bleeding.

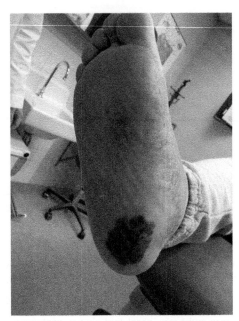

Fig. 10. Acral lentiginous melanoma: an asymmetric, brown-black macule with color variation and irregular borders that presents on the palms, soles, and nails.

Investigation of the skin is based on the ABCDE criteria for changing moles to identify asymmetry, border irregularity, color abnormalities, diameter greater than 6 mm, and an evolving nature that serve as warning signs of melanoma development.[54] Change in color, shape, or size over the course of months is the most sensitive clinical sign for melanoma; this highlights the importance of full-body skin examinations, including self-skin examinations, to detect melanocytic lesions that can arise on any cutaneous surface. Dermoscopy (requires a fluid interface and a hand-held lens-stereomicroscope-digital imaging system that makes direct skin contact) is occasionally used to differentiate between early melanoma stages and benign lesions.[55] High-risk individuals often warrant photographically assisted evaluation to document the progression of lesions over time.[56] However, pathology is the gold standard for diagnosis including architectural pattern and histology. Any suspicious lesion should be biopsied, ideally using excisional biopsy. Because melanoma has a high risk of metastasis, examination of lymph node basins and an abdominal examination to look for hepatosplenomegaly are crucial components of the examination. Routine imaging studies and blood work have shown limited value in the initial evaluation of asymptomatic patients with cutaneous melanoma 4 mm in diameter or less. However, patients with stage III and IV melanoma warrant an initial positron emission tomography scan, followed by chest, pelvis, and abdominal computed tomographic scans and/or brain magnetic resonance imaging to identify metastatic spread.[57] The biopsy report for cutaneous melanoma should include the tumor thickness (Breslow depth), ulceration, dermal mitotic rate (number of mitoses/mm^2), presence of microsatellites, and anatomic level of invasion.[58] Breslow depth of invasion is the strongest predictor of survival with increased depth of invasion associated with a worse prognosis than a shallow lesion.[59] Sentinel lymph node biopsy (SLNB), an invaluable technique for staging and prognosis, uses lymphoscintigraphy to identify the "sentinel" or first cancer-infected node in the regional basis. SLNB provides accurate information regarding subclinical node status with minimal morbidity, is cost-effective, and allows for appropriate administration of adjuvant therapy if indicated.

Staging

Current melanoma staging uses the tumor-node-metastasis staging system introduced by the American Joint Committee on Cancer in 2000.[60] Under this system, T staging is determined by the Breslow depth, N staging by micro or macro nodal metastasis, and M staging by organ metastasis. Prognosis depends on the melanoma stage at diagnosis, because the involvement of regional lymph nodes or distant metastases is associated with an increasingly worse prognosis. Localized melanoma (TxNoMo) is associated with a 5-year survival rate between 61% and 100% depending on tumor thickness and ulceration.[54] The prognosis of locally invasive melanoma (TxNxMo) depends on the number of involved lymph nodes and tumor burden. Five-year survival rates range from 40% to 78%. Invasive melanoma (TxNxMx) generally has a poor prognosis with 5-year survival rates less than 20% and is highly dependent on where the melanoma has metastasized.[54]

Treatment

Surgery is the primary treatment for localized melanoma. Standard efficacious margins for excision have yet to be determined. Numerous studies have determined that 5 mm margins for melanoma in situ, 1 cm margins for melanoma less than or equal to 1 mm in depth, and 2 cm margins for melanoma of intermediate thickness (1–4 mm Breslow depth) are effective in preventing local disease recurrence.[61] As previously mentioned, sentinel lymph node biopsy is a technique routinely indicated for melanoma greater than or equal to 1 mm in depth and/or exhibiting features of poor prognosis including ulceration, lymphovascular invasion, and mitotic rate greater than or equal to $1/mm^2$. If micrometastases are discovered on the sentinel lymph node biopsy, a complete lymph node dissection is necessary. The sentinel biopsy serves as an important cornerstone in melanoma treatment and prognosis of survival.[62] Numerous adjuvant therapies are currently under investigation for melanoma treatment, including immunotherapy agents, biologic response modifiers, and melanoma vaccines. However, no survival benefit has been demonstrated for adjuvant chemotherapy, nonspecific (passive) immunotherapy (including interferon), radiation therapy, retinoid therapy, vitamin therapy, or biologic therapy.[63]

Prognosis

The 5-year survival rate for people whose melanoma is detected and treated before it spreads to the lymph nodes is 98%, and the 5-year survival rates for regional and distant stage melanomas are 62% and 16%, respectively.[21] Melanoma survivors have an approximately 9-fold increased risk of developing another melanoma compared with the general population.[64] Individuals who have a history of melanoma should have a full-body examination at least every 3 months and perform regular self-examinations for new and changing moles. Public health campaigns over the past 2 decades promoting skin care, education regarding sun exposure, and earlier detection have led to an increased number of diagnoses of thin melanomas with a better prognosis than more advanced-stage, thick lesions.[65]

Prevention

Limitation of sun exposure serves as the primary prevention of melanoma.[53] Sunscreen has been the only truly effective public health measure to decrease sun exposure. Strategies such as decreasing midday outdoor activities and recommendation of wide-brimmed hats and long-sleeved clothing have not been widely accepted by the general public. There has been increasing debate over the past decade over prior studies associating increased melanoma risk with sunscreen use. It is important for health professionals to inform patients that these earlier studies failed to account for confounding factors, used sunscreens that were not broad-spectrum (important because melanoma is particularly susceptible to UVA), and sunscreen was generally not appropriately applied.[54]

COMMON BENIGN SKIN LESIONS

In addition to skin cancer, several common benign skin lesions should be familiar to health care providers in any field including seborrheic keratosis, sebaceous hyperplasia, solar lentigo, melanocytic nevi, milia, and venous lakes.

Seborrheic Keratosis

Seborrheic keratosis is a common, wart-like pigmented tumor (**Fig. 11**). The lesion appears as a smooth, flat, waxy plaque with a color that varies from tan to dark brown. The pathogenesis of seborrheic keratosis is unknown, but on histology, it appears as an exophytic growth of the epidermis. The growth is commonly identified as a horn of pseudocysts filled with keratin. These lesions typically grow in crops on the trunk, face, and extremities. They commonly present after the age of 40 years but can occasionally occur earlier in life. A rare subtype of seborrheic keratosis is dermatosis papulosa nigra, which manifests as heavily pigmented, small papules on the cheeks of darker skin types. Treatment of seborrheic keratosis is not necessary because of their benign nature; however, curettage, cryotherapy with liquid nitrogen, dermabrasion, and laser therapy have been used to remove the lesions for cosmetic reasons.

Sebaceous Hyperplasia

Sebaceous hyperplasia represents one of the most common sebaceous lesions found on the skin (**Fig. 12**). It is an accumulation of enlarged but otherwise normal sebaceous glands around a central follicle. These are usually seen on the face as rosettes of yellow, tiny papules with a central dell just beneath the skin surface. No therapy is needed for sebaceous hyperplasia because the lesions are simply a cosmetic phenomenon. Treatment includes electrodesiccation and laser ablation. They can often resemble BCCs; so a biopsy may be needed if a question of origin exists.

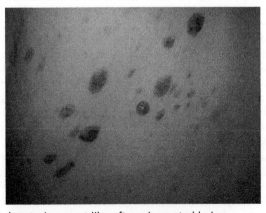

Fig. 11. Seborrheic keratosis: a wart-like often pigmented lesion.

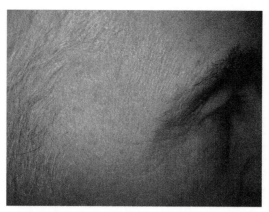

Fig. 12. Sebaceous hyperplasia: yellow papules in rosettes with telangiectasias.

Solar Lentigo

Solar lentigo, also known as age spots or liver spots, are common acquired lesions in older adults (**Fig. 13**). They appear as multiple, tan-brown macules with irregular shape. Solar lentigo is commonly found on sun-exposed areas, especially the back of the hands, face, and scalp. Histologic examination demonstrates an increased layer of pigment in the basal layer of the epidermis but no increase in melanocytes or nests. Solar lentigo is a cosmetic problem that simply warrants periodic monitoring for pigment change and darkening. If so desired, lesions can be treated with liquid nitrogen or laser therapy.

Melanocytic Nevi

Melanocytic nevi are benign neoplasms that are composed of the pigment producing cells called melanocytes (**Fig. 14**). They represent the most common human tumor in the world. Virtually, everyone will develop at least one "mole" throughout their lifetime. These lesions are benign, first appear around the age of 2 to 3 years, and typically stabilize around the age of 30 to 40 years. The number of moles on an individual is related to degree of skin pigmentation. It is now recognized that acquired melanocytic nevi are induced by certain trigger factors such as the sun and hormones. Genetic

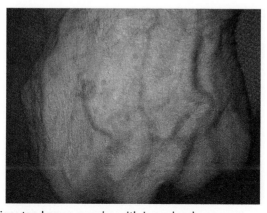

Fig. 13. Solar lentigo: tan-brown macules with irregular shape.

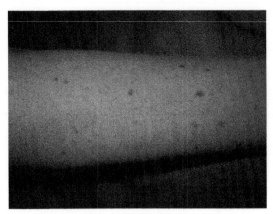

Fig. 14. Nevi: brown-tan macules with regular borders.

factors are also especially seen in various familial conditions. Lesions commonly begin as tan macules, which can evolve into darker papules. Color varies from tan, red, brown, dark brown, or skin-colored, but they are usually a stable color and shape. Nevi that appear greater than 1 cm in diameter suggest a congenital rather than an acquired melanocytic nevus. They often appear on the face, trunk, and extremities of light-skinned individuals. In dark-skinned individuals, acral melanocytic nevi are more common.[66]

Acquired nevi should be monitored clinically for atypia and evolution into dysplastic nevi. Dysplastic nevi often have an irregularity to their pigmentation and are usually larger than nevi. Some have a "fried egg" appearance and can be numerous on the trunk and extremities. Regular skin examinations, surgical excision of the severely dysplastic nevi, and photodocumentation are used as treatment options. Several prospective studies have demonstrated that patients with dysplastic nevi have an increased risk of developing melanoma.[67]

Milia

Milia are tiny variants of epidermoid cysts that usually favor the face, especially the cheeks, temples, and periorbital regions (**Fig. 15**). Each lesion is a 1 to 2 mm,

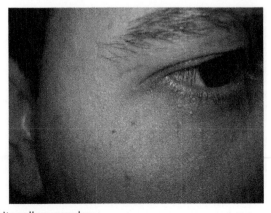

Fig. 15. Milia: white-yellow papules.

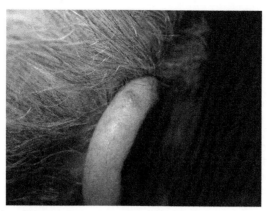

Fig. 16. Venous lake: dilated vessel on the skin surface.

dome-shaped, white-yellow plaque that is filled with keratin. Milia can be primary or secondary, following trauma or dermabrasion. Treatment consists of incision and expression of the keratin contents.

Venous Lake

"Venous lake" is a term used to describe a dilated blood vessel on the skin surface (**Fig. 16**). These lesions are compressible, dome-shaped, blue-pink nodules that are commonly found on the lip or ears. Because venous lakes can appear violaceous in color, they are sometimes mistaken for melanoma. However, the compressible nature of venous lakes indicates a vascular origin instead of a neoplasm. Therapy is by excision or laser ablation.

SUMMARY

This article serves as an introduction to skin cancer and benign skin lesions for dental professionals. By simply becoming aware of common lesions and their phenotypic presentation, dental professionals are empowered to detect suspicious lesions in unaware patients and subsequently refer them to a dermatologist for evaluation. Skin lesions are extremely common, and early detection of dangerous lesions makes skin cancer one of the most highly curable malignancies. Dentists can have an impact on the health of their patients by examining the skin, making the appropriate referral, and following up with the patient to determine if they have seen a dermatologist.

REFERENCES

1. Bolognia JL, Jorizzo JL, Schaffer JV. Dermatology. 2nd edition. St. Louis (MO): Elsevier; 2011.
2. Basal cell carcinoma. Skin Cancer Foundation. http://www.skincancer.org/skin-cancer-information/skin-cancer-facts#general. Accessed September 2012.
3. Rogers HW, Weinstock MA, Harris AR, et al. Incidence estimate of nonmelanoma skin cancer in the United States. Arch Dermatol 2010;146(3):283–7.
4. Lear JT, Smith AG. Basal cell carcinoma. Postgrad Med J 1997;73:538–42.
5. Christenson LJ, Borrowman TA, Vachon CM, et al. Incidence of basal cell and squamous cell carcinomas in a population younger than 40 years. JAMA 2005; 294(6):681–90.

6. Skin cancer statistics. American Academy of Dermatology. http://www.aad.org/media-resources/stats-and-facts/conditions/skin-cancer. Accessed September 2012.

7. Marcil I, Stern R. Risk of developing subsequent NMSC in patients with a history of NMSc: a critical review of the literature and metaanalysis. Arch Dermatol 2000; 136:1524–30.

8. Saladi RN, Persaud AN. The causes of skin cancer: a comprehensive review. Drugs Today (Barc) 2005;41(1):37–53.

9. Gallagher RP, Hill GB, Bajdik CD, et al. Sunlight exposure, pigmentary factors, and risk of nonmelanocytic skin cancer. I: basal cell carcinoma. Arch Dermatol 1995;131(2):157–63.

10. Corona R, Dogliotti E, Eric M, et al. Risk factors for basal cell carcinoma in a Mediterranean population: role of recreational sun exposure early in life. Arch Dermatol 2001;137:1162–8.

11. Kricker A, Armstrong BK, English DR, et al. Does intermittent sun exposure cause basal cell carcinoma? A case-control study in Western Australia. Int J Cancer 1995;60:489–94.

12. Lear JT, Tan BB, Smith AG, et al. Risk factors for basal cell carcinoma in the UK: case-control study in 806 patients. J R Soc Med 1997;90:371–4.

13. Ron E. Cancer risks from medical radiation. Health Phys 2003;85(1):47–59.

14. Yu HS, Liao WT, Chai CY. Arsenic carcinogenesis in the skin. J Biomed Sci 2006; 13(5):657–66.

15. Ho WL, Murphy GM. Update on the pathogenesis of post-transplant skin cancer in renal transplant recipients. Br J Dermatol 2008;158(2):217–24.

16. Nijsten TE, Stern RS. The increased risk of skin cancer is persistent after discontinuation of psoralen+ultraviolet A: a cohort study. J Invest Dermatol 2003;121: 252–8.

17. Sasson M, Mallory SB. Malignant primary skin tumors in children. Curr Opin Pediatr 1996;8(4):372–7.

18. Hartevelt M, Bavinck J, Koote A, et al. Incidence of skin cancer after renal transplantation in the Netherlands. Transplantation 1990;49:506–9.

19. Orengo I, Brown T, Rosen T. Cutaneous neoplasia in organ transplant recipients. Curr Probl Dermatol 1999;11:123–58.

20. Cancer facts and figures 2008. American Cancer Society. http://www.cancer.org/Research/CancerFactsFigures/cancer-facts-figures-2008. Accessed September 2012.

21. Cancer facts and figures 2011. American Cancer Society. http://www.cancer.org/Research/CancerFactsFigures/CancerFactsFigures/cancer-facts-figures-2011. Accessed September 2012.

22. Barksdale SK, O'Connor N, Barnhill R. Prognostic factors for cutaneous squamous cell and basal cell carcinoma: determinants of risk of recurrence, metastasis, and development of subsequent skin cancers. Surg Oncol Clin N Am 1997;6(3):625–38.

23. Roewert-Huber J, Lange-Asschenfeldt B, Stockfleth E, et al. Epidemiology and aetiology of basal cell carcinoma. Br J Dermatol 2007;157(2):47–51.

24. Braun RP, Klumb F, Girard C, et al. Three-dimensional reconstruction of basal cell carcinomas. Dermatol Surg 2005;31(5):562–6.

25. Owens DM, Watt FM. Contribution of stem cells and differentiated cells to epidermal tumours. Nat Rev Cancer 2003;3(6):444–51.

26. Hutchin M. Sustained Hedgehog signaling is required for basal cell carcinoma proliferation and survival: conditional skin tumorigenesis recapitulates the hair growth cycle. Genes Dev 2005;19:214–23.

27. Scrivener Y, Grosshans E, Cribier B. Variations of basal cell carcinomas according to gender, age, location and histopathological subtype. Br J Dermatol 2002; 147:41–7.
28. Batra RS, Kelley LC. Predictors of extensive subclinical spread in nonmelanoma skin cancer treated with Mohs micrographic surgery. Arch Dermatol 2002;138: 1043–51.
29. Rowe D. Comparison of treatment modalities for basal cell carcinoma. Clin Dermatol 1995;13:617–20.
30. Walling HW, Fosko SW, Geraminejad PA, et al. Aggressive basal cell carcinoma: presentation, pathogenesis, and management. Cancer Metastasis Rev 2004;23: 389–402.
31. Malone JP, Fedok FG, Belchis DA, et al. Basal cell carcinoma metastatic to the parotid: report of a new case and review of the literature. Ear Nose Throat J 2000;79(7):511–5, 518–9.
32. Ting P, Kasper R, Arlette J. Metastatic basal cell carcinoma: report of two cases and literature review. J Cutan Med Surg 2005;9:10–5.
33. Kwa RE, Campana K, Moy RL. Biology of cutaneous squamous cell carcinoma. J Am Acad Dermatol 1992;26:1–26.
34. Miller DL, Weinstock MA. Nonmelanoma skin cancer in the United States: incidence. J Am Acad Dermatol 1994;30:774–8.
35. Gallagher RP, Hill GB, Bajdik CD, et al. Sunlight exposure, pigmentation factors, and risk of nonmelanocytic skin cancer. II. Squamous cell carcinoma. Arch Dermatol 1995;131:164–9.
36. Fuchs A, Marmur E. The kinetics of skin cancer. Dermatol Surg 2007;33:1099.
37. Salasche S. Epidemiology of actinic keratoses and squamous cell carcinoma. J Am Acad Dermatol 2000;42:4–7.
38. Alam M, Ratner D. SCC. N Engl J Med 2001;344:975–83.
39. Johnson TM, Rowe DE, Nelson BR, et al. Squamous cell carcinoma of the skin (excluding lip and oral mucosa). J Am Acad Dermatol 1992;26:467–84.
40. Rowe DE, Carroll RJ, Day CL Jr. Prognostic factors for local recurrence, metastasis, and survival rates in squamous cell carcinoma of the skin, ear, and lip: implications for treatment modality selection. J Am Acad Dermatol 1992;26:976–90.
41. Abide J, Nahai F, Bennett R. The meaning of surgical margins. Plast Reconstr Surg 1984;73(3):492–7.
42. Neville J, Welch E, Leffell D. Management of NMSC in 2007. Nature 2007;4(8): 462–9.
43. Smeets N. Little evidence available on treatments for basal cell carcinoma. Cancer Treat Rev 2005;31:143–6.
44. Linos E, Swetter S, Cockburn MG, et al. Increasing burden of melanoma in the United States. J Invest Dermatol 2009;129(7):1666–74.
45. Cancer epidemiology in older adolescents & young adults. SEER AYA Monograph 2007;53–7.
46. Rigel DS, Russak J, Friedman R. The evolution of melanoma diagnosis: 25 years beyond the ABCDs. CA Cancer J Clin 2010;60(5):301–16.
47. Demierre MF, Nathanson L. Chemoprevention of melanoma: an unexplored strategy. J Clin Oncol 2003;21(1):158–65.
48. Williams ML, Sagebiel RW. Melanoma risk factors and atypical moles. West J Med 1994;160(4):343–50.
49. Elder DE, Clark WH Jr, Elenitsas R, et al. The early and intermediate precursor lesions of tumor progression in the melanocytic system: common acquired nevi and atypical (dysplastic) nevi. Semin Diagn Pathol 1993;10:18–35.

50. Maldonado JL, Fridlyand J, Patel H, et al. Determinants of BRAF mutations in primary melanomas. J Natl Cancer Inst 2003;95(24):1878–90.
51. Yang G, Rajadurai A, Tsao H. Recurrent patterns of dual RB and p53 pathway inactivation in melanoma. J Invest Dermatol 2005;125:1242–51.
52. Autier P. Perspectives in melanoma prevention: the case of sunbeds. Eur J Cancer 2004;40:2367–76.
53. Ting W, Schultz K, Cac NN, et al. Tanning bed exposure increases the risk of malignant melanoma. Int J Dermatol 2007;46(12):1253–7.
54. Abbasi NR, Shaw HM, Rigel DS, et al. Early diagnosis of cutaneous melanoma: revisiting the ABCD criteria. JAMA 2004;292(22):2771–6.
55. Massone C, Di Stefani A, Soyer HP. Dermoscopy for skin cancer detection. Curr Opin Oncol 2005;17:147–53.
56. Halpern AC. Total body skin imaging as an aid to melanoma detection. Semin Cutan Med Surg 2003;22:2–8.
57. Miranda EP, Gertner M, Wall J, et al. Routine imaging of asymptomatic melanoma patients with metastasis to sentinel lymph nodes rarely identifies systemic disease. Arch Surg 2004;139(8):831–7.
58. Bichakjian CK, Halpern AC, Johnson TM, et al. Guidelines of care for the management of primary cutaneous melanoma. J Am Acad Dermatol 2011; 65(5):1032–47.
59. Clark WH Jr, Elder DE, Guerry D 4th, et al. Model predicting survival in stage I melanoma based on tumor progression. J Natl Cancer Inst 1989;81(24): 1893–904.
60. Balch CM, Buzaid AC, Atkins MB, et al. A new American Joint Committee on Cancer staging system for cutaneous melanoma. Cancer 2000;88(6):1484–91.
61. Kunishige JH, Brodland DG, Zitelli JA. Surgical margins for melanoma in situ. J Am Acad Dermatol 2012;66(3):438–44.
62. Gershenwald JE, Thompson W, Mansfield PF, et al. Multi-institutional melanoma lymphatic mapping experience: the prognostic value of sentinel lymph node status in 612 stage I or II melanoma patients. J Clin Oncol 1999;17(3):976–83.
63. Veronesi U, Adamus J, Aubert C, et al. A randomized trial of adjuvant chemo-therapy and immunotherapy in cutaneous melanoma. N Engl J Med 1982; 307(15):913–6.
64. Bradford PT, Freedman DM, Goldstein AM, et al. Increased risk of second primary cancers after a diagnosis of melanoma. Arch Dermatol 2010;146(3):265–72.
65. Parkin DM, Bray F, Ferlay J, et al. Global cancer statistics, 2002. CA Cancer J Clin 2005;55(2):74–108.
66. Palicka GA, Rhodes AR. Acral melanocytic nevi: prevalence and distribution of gross morphologic features in white and black adults. Arch Dermatol 2010; 146(10):1085–94.
67. Kraemer KH, Greene MH. Dysplastic nevi and cutaneous melanoma. Lancet 1983;2(8358):1076–7.

Nutrition and Physical Activity in Health Promotion and Disease Prevention

Potential Role for the Dental Profession

Sharon R. Akabas, PhD*, Joanne D. Chouinard, DMD, MPH, MS, Bonnie R. Bernstein, PhD

KEYWORDS

- Nutrition • Physical activity • Oral health • Lifestyle • Obesity • Metabolic syndrome
- Chronic disease prevention • Diabetes • De novo lipogenesis

KEY POINTS

- Nutrition contributes to at least 6 of the 10 leading causes of death in the United States, yet less than one-third of dental students feel competent to discuss the relationship of nutrition and systemic disease with their patients.
- The American Dental Association policy statements acknowledge a need for health professionals and organizations to provide continuing education to professionals and counseling to patients to combat the growing problems of overweight and obesity. Dentists can play a major role in educating patients to adopt a healthier lifestyle, including nutrition and physical activity recommendations. In addition, an understanding of the complexity of behavior change may enhance the dentist's ability to assist their patients in making desired changes.
- The interaction of general health and oral health is seen most clearly in the interaction between diabetes and periodontal health, each potentially affecting the other in a downward spiral of worsening general health.
- Because the current nutrition and activity behaviors of most Americans is far from optimal, much can be gained as dentists develop a better understanding of the difficulties of sustained behavior change and become proficient in counseling approaches that lead to improved oral health for patients.

INTRODUCTION

Nutrition contributes to at least 6 of the 10 leading causes of death in the United States,[1] and less than one-third of dental students feel competent to speak about nutrition with their patients.[2] Cardiovascular disease is the leading cause of death in

Department of Pediatrics, Institute of Human Nutrition, Columbia University Medical Center, 168th Street, New York, NY 10032, USA
* Corresponding author. Institute of Human Nutrition, 630 West 168th Street, PH 15-1512, New York, NY 10032.
E-mail address: sa109@columbia.edu

Dent Clin N Am 56 (2012) 791–808
http://dx.doi.org/10.1016/j.cden.2012.07.006
0011-8532/12/$ – see front matter Published by Elsevier Inc.

dental.theclinics.com

the United States, accounting for one in three deaths.[3] The American Heart Association has identified seven modifiable health parameters known to reduce the risk of cardiovascular disease, yet only about 2% of adults in the United States engage in the lifestyle behaviors that allow possession of all seven.[4] These health parameters include not smoking; being physically active; having normal blood pressure, blood glucose, total cholesterol levels, and normal weight; and eating a healthy diet. Other articles in this issue deal with smoking, blood pressure, obesity, and diabetes; this article provides the scientific bases of key nutrition and physical activity recommendations. Most of the American Heart Association recommendations are currently not being met,[4] and substantial behavior changes are required to help patients reach desired goals. This represents an important opportunity for dentists to play a role in improving their patients overall health. A brief section describes some of the underlying reasons that patients do not comply with recommendations, even when it is in their own best interests to do so. We also include guidelines in the use of active listening and motivational interviewing (MI), where the practitioner collaborates with the patient to make desired lifestyle changes.

NUTRITION AND ORAL HEALTH

In young children and adolescents, dentists are very aware of the outcome of constant local exposure of teeth to free sugars, sticky refined carbohydrates, and highly processed foods.[5] Despite 50 years of water fluoridation[6] and decades of nutrition advice, pediatric dentists in the United States are alarmed by caries increase in very young children.[7] Young children are routinely admitted to hospital operating rooms in the United States with the need for general anesthesia to treat multiple decayed and infected teeth.[8] Parents seem disconnected from the relationship of a food environment filled with sweets, constant sipping of fruit juice and sugar-sweetened beverages (SSBs), choosing bottled water over fluoridated tap water, and their lack of reinforcement of brushing of teeth, contributing to their child's dental caries.[8]

Developing countries adopting the lifestyle and dietary patterns of Western countries have increased caries incidence, with few healthcare resources to treat the pathology.[5] The evolving global food environment is a worldwide public health hazard, replete with a highly processed, inexpensive, ubiquitous supply of high caloric density and low nutrient density foods. The dismal Western dietary pattern, illustrated in **Table 1**[9] from the 2010 dietary guidelines on current US consumption patterns, coupled with the sedentary habits of most of the population, has contributed to 66% of adults being overweight and 35.7% of US adults being obese in 2010.[10] Obesity contributes to symptoms of metabolic syndrome with frequent clustering of insulin resistance, ectopic hepatic fat,[11] increased visceral fat,[11] and chronic low-grade inflammation called "metaflammation."[12] Notably, metaflammation is common to all inflammatory diseases including atherosclerosis, rheumatoid arthritis, inflammatory bowel disease, asthma, diabetes, and periodontitis.[11,13]

The dentist may be less aware of how lifestyle interventions beyond smoking cessation, such as physical activity and diet, mitigate chronic illness.[14,15] The same child presenting with rampant dental caries who is overweight or obese becomes an adolescent at risk for nonalcoholic fatty liver disease,[11] atherosclerotic cardiovascular disease, and type 2 diabetes mellitus.[16]

The American Dental Association (ADA) policy statements acknowledge a need for health professionals and organizations to provide continuing education to professionals and counseling to patients to combat the growing problems of overweight and obesity.[17] Information defining the relationships between oral health and nutrition,

Table 1
Top 25 sources of calories among Americans ages 2 years and older, NHANES 2005–2006[a]

Rank	Overall, Ages 2+ Years (mean kcal/d; total daily calories = 2157)	Children and Adolescents, Ages 2–18 Years (mean kcal/d; total daily calories = 2027)	Adults and Older Adults, Ages 19+ Years (mean kcal/d; total daily calories = 2199)
1	Grain-based desserts[b] (138 kcal)	Grain-based desserts (138 kcal)	Grain-based desserts (138 kcal)
2	Yeast breads[c] (129 kcal)	Pizza (136 kcal)	Yeast breads (134 kcal)
3	Chicken and chicken mixed dishes[d] (121 kcal)	Soda/energy/sports drinks (118 kcal)	Chicken and chicken mixed dishes (123 kcal)
4	Soda/energy/sports drinks[e] (114 kcal)	Yeast breads (114 kcal)	Soda/energy/sports drinks (112 kcal)
5	Pizza (98 kcal)	Chicken and chicken mixed dishes (113 kcal)	Alcoholic beverages (106 kcal)
6	Alcoholic beverages (82 kcal)	Pasta and pasta dishes (91 kcal)	Pizza (86 kcal)
7	Pasta and pasta dishes[f] (81 kcal)	Reduced-fat milk (86 kcal)	Tortillas, burritos, tacos (85 kcal)
8	Tortillas, burritos, tacos[g] (80 kcal)	Dairy desserts (76 kcal)	Pasta and pasta dishes (78 kcal)
9	Beef and beef mixed dishes[h] (64 kcal)	Potato/corn/other chips (70 kcal)	Beef and beef mixed dishes (71 kcal)
10	Dairy desserts[i] (62 kcal)	Ready-to-eat cereals (65 kcal)	Dairy desserts (58 kcal)
11	Potato/corn/other chips (56 kcal)	Tortillas, burritos, tacos (63 kcal)	Burgers (53 kcal)
12	Burgers (53 kcal)	Whole milk (60 kcal)	Regular cheese (51 kcal)
13	Reduced-fat milk (51 kcal)	Candy (56 kcal)	Potato/corn/other chips (51 kcal)
14	Regular cheese (49 kcal)	Fruit drinks (55 kcal)	Sausage, franks, bacon, and ribs (49 kcal)
15	Ready-to-eat cereals (49 kcal)	Burgers (55 kcal)	Nuts/seeds and nut/seed mixed dishes (47 kcal)
16	Sausage, franks, bacon, and ribs (49 kcal)	Fried white potatoes (52 kcal)	Fried white potatoes (46 kcal)
17	Fried white potatoes (48 kcal)	Sausage, franks, bacon, and ribs (47 kcal)	Ready-to-eat cereals (44 kcal)
18	Candy (47 kcal)	Regular cheese (43 kcal)	Candy (44 kcal)
19	Nuts/seeds and nut/seed mixed dishes[j] (42 kcal)	Beef and beef mixed dishes (43 kcal)	Eggs and egg mixed dishes (42 kcal)
20	Eggs and egg mixed dishes[k] (39 kcal)	100% fruit juice, not orange/grapefruit (35 kcal)	Rice and rice mixed dishes (41 kcal)
21	Rice and rice mixed dishes[l] (36 kcal)	Eggs and egg mixed dishes (30 kcal)	Reduced-fat milk (39 kcal)
22	Fruit drinks[m] (36 kcal)	Pancakes, waffles, and French toast (29 kcal)	Quick breads (36 kcal)

(continued on next page)

Rank	Overall, Ages 2+ Years (mean kcal/d; total daily calories = 2157)	Children and Adolescents, Ages 2–18 Years (mean kcal/d; total daily calories = 2027)	Adults and Older Adults, Ages 19+ Years (mean kcal/d; total daily calories = 2199)
		Table 1 *(continued)*	
23	Whole milk (33 kcal)	Crackers (28 kcal)	Other fish and fish mixed dishes[n] (30 kcal)
24	Quick breads[o] (32 kcal)	Nuts/seeds and nut/seed mixed dishes (27 kcal)	Fruit drinks (29 kcal)
25	Cold cuts (27 kcal)	Cold cuts (24 kcal)	Salad dressing (29 kcal)

[a] Data are drawn from analyses of usual dietary intakes conducted by the National Cancer Institute. Foods and beverages consumed were divided into 97 categories and ranked according to calorie contribution to the diet. Table shows each food category and its mean calorie contribution for each age group. Additional information on calorie contribution by age, gender, and race/ethnicity is available at http://riskfactor.cancer.gov/diet/foodsources/.
[b] Includes cake, cookies, pie cobbler, sweet rolls pastries, and donuts.
[c] Includes white bread or rolls, mixed-grain bread, flavored bread, whole-wheat bread, and bagels.
[d] Includes fried or baked chicken parts and chicken strips/patties, chicken stir-fries, chicken casseroles, chicken sandwiches, chicken salads, stewed chicken, and other chicken mixed dishes.
[e] Sodas, energy drinks, sports drinks, and sweetened bottled water including vitamin water.
[f] Includes macaroni and cheese, spaghetti, other pasta with or without sauces, filled pasta (eg, lasagna and ravioli), and noodles.
[g] Also includes nachos, quesadillas, and other Mexican mixed dishes.
[h] Includes steak, meatloaf, beef with noodles, and beef stew.
[i] Includes ice cream, frozen yogurt, sherbet, milk shakes, and pudding.
[j] Includes peanut butter, peanuts, and mixed nuts.
[k] Includes scrambled eggs, omelets, fried eggs, egg breakfast sandwiches/biscuits, boiled and poached eggs, egg salad, deviled eggs, quiche, and egg substitutes.
[l] Includes white rice, Spanish rice, and fried rice.
[m] Includes fruit-flavored drinks, fruit juice drinks, and fruit punch.
[n] Fish other than tuna or shrimp.
[o] Includes muffins, biscuits, and cornbread.
Data from National Cancer Institute food sources of energy among U.S. population, 2005–2006. Risk factor monitoring and methods. Control and population sciences. National Cancer Institute; 2010. Available at: http://riskfactor.cancer.gov/diet/foodsources/. Updated May 21, 2010. Accessed May 21, 2010.

and systemic and oral health are to be incorporated into documents and educational materials.[18]

The 2010 dietary guidelines provide a focal point of what every dentist should know to meet ADA policy guidelines and global public health challenges of oral and systemic health interactions. The 2010 Guidelines center on unprocessed whole foods that are nutrient dense but energy poor per kilocalorie consumed.[9] This eating style features minimally processed foods and avoids manufactured food products. It emphasizes whole grains, fruits, vegetables, and foods high in long-chain omega 3 polyunsaturated fat. It stresses reducing saturated fats, moderate alcohol intake, decreasing SSBs, reducing refined grains, and avoidance of trans fat.[19] The whole grains, fruits, and vegetables provide fiber[20] and promote satiety.[21] Protein sources and consumption are adequate in the United States and there is a recommendation to seek lean sources of protein and add vegetable protein sources, such as nuts and legumes.[9]

Ludwig[19] emphasizes that traditional diets, such as the "Mediterranean diet," incorporate most of the protective aspects of the guidelines, such as minimal processing with little refined carbohydrates, and have low added sugar content. Traditional diets from such countries as Japan and China exemplify the dietary guidelines with frequency and variety of fruits and vegetables as the cornerstones of healthy food choices. They are easy to follow for those ethnic groups accustomed to them.[22]

In comparison, the food consumed in the Western diet, built on fast food, partially hydrogenated added fats, refined carbohydrates, and added sugars has high caloric density with dismal nutritional value.[9] The number one food category is grain-based desserts, which are refined grain foods with added fats, including cakes, cookies, pie, cobbler, sweet rolls, pastries, and donuts (see **Table 1**).[9]

The most relevant points in the guidelines for dentists include:

- *Increase intake of whole grains, vegetables, and fruits*: A diet high in whole grains, fruits, and vegetables has a great deal of volume and provides satiety.[21] This contributes to what is described in the guidelines as "moderate" scientific evidence that adults who eat more whole grains, particularly those higher in dietary fiber, have a lower body weight compared with adults who eat very few whole grains.[9]
- *Reduce intake of SSBs*: This recommendation stresses that SSBs provide calories and little nutrients, displace foods of nutrient density, and should be considered only after nutrient needs have been fulfilled but calorie limits have not been met.[9] Given the universal availability of these beverages, emphasis that constant exposure to these liquids increases caries risk, and the calories increase obesity risk,[20] should be part of preventive care.
- *Monitor intake of 100% fruit juice for children and adolescents, especially those who are overweight or obese*: Natural sugars are as cariogenic as free or added sugars.[9] Patients may have difficulty distinguishing 100% real fruit juice from juice drink. Food manufacturers place juice content in small print on the back of the nutrition label. Front labels often show the product provides 100% of a nutrient, such as "provides 100% Daily Value for vitamin C" in larger print. This is confusing for patients with limited English language skills and makes a wise purchase more challenging. Unless the package also states it is "100% juice," it is not 100% juice. Sweetened juice products are considerably cheaper but are SSBs rather than fruit juice, and should be avoided.[9]
- *Monitor calorie intake from alcoholic beverages for adults*: Moderate consumption of alcohol, thought to be cardioprotective, is defined as one glass of wine per day (5 oz) for women and two glasses (10 oz) for men. Greater amounts than this are associated with weight gain.[9]
- *Milk and milk products*: Dentists are familiar with recommendations for calcium and vitamin D intakes for healthy teeth, periodontium, and bones,[23] and recommend milk, cheese, and yogurt to patients as sources of calcium. However, evidence in adults and children indicates that consumption of milk and milk products does not play a special role in weight management.[9] Added fats, sugars, and excessive portion sizes remain embedded in the Western diet and patients should be mindful of portion size and fat content when choosing calcium-rich foods.

The Dietary Approaches to Stop Hypertension (DASH) Diet and the Therapeutic Lifestyle Changes (TLC) diets are specialized, but in many ways similar, to the 2010 guidelines. DASH is formulated to reduce hypertension,[24] and TLC focuses on reducing low-density lipoprotein to ease metabolic syndrome and coronary heart disease.[25] A summary and description of DASH and TLC are found in **Table 2**[24] and **Table 3**.[25]

Table 2	
DASH diet total consumption guidelines for the DASH diet	
Fruits and vegetables	4.5 cups per day
Fiber-rich whole grains	3 1-oz-equivalent servings per day
Sodium	<1500 mg per day
Sugar sweetened beverages	<450 kcal (36 oz) per wk
Supplemented with:	
Nuts/legumes/seeds	>4 1-oz servings per wk
Saturated fat	<7% of total energy intake
Processed meats	None or <2 servings per wk

Data from United States Department of Health and Human Services, National Institutes of Health, National Heart Lung and Blood Institute. Publication No. 06–4082. Your guide to lowering your blood pressure with DASH. Available at: http://www.nhlbi.nih.gov/health/public/heart/hbp/dash/new_dash.pdf. Accessed March 30, 2012.

MyPlate.gov (**Fig. 1**)[26] and My Plate Planner (**Fig. 2**)[27] are visual tools that reflect the message of what consumers should place on their plates. A 9-in plate replaces an 11-in plate to encourage smaller portion selection and promotes increasing the amount, and frequency, of fruit and vegetable consumption. My Plate Planner,[27] from the New York City Department of Health, may be more effective in encouraging compliance because a full half of each lunch and dinner plate is filled with low starch (low glycemic load) and low caloric density vegetables. The average US consumer adopting this practice would greatly improve their consumption patterns. No whole fruit or a single vegetable, except fried potatoes, are noted in the top 25 foods most frequently consumed in the United States from the 2005 to 2006 NHANES Data (see **Table 1**).[9] Smaller areas, one-quarter of the plate for protein and one-quarter of the plate for carbohydrate, comprise the other half of plate contents.

Table 3	
TLC diet guidelines	
Limits	
Saturated fat	<7% of calories
Total fat	<25%–35% of daily calories from total fat (including saturated fat calories)
Other low-density lipoprotein lowering strategies:	
	2 g per day of plant stanols or sterols
	10–25 g per day of soluble fiber
	Consume enough calories to reach or maintain a healthy weight
	30 min of a moderate-intensity physical activity, such as brisk walking, on most and preferably all days of the wk

Data from Centers for Disease Control and Prevention. Can lifestyle modifications using therapeutic lifestyle changes (TLC) reduce weight and the risk for chronic disease? Available at: www.cdc.gov/nutrition/downloads/R2P_life_change.pdf. Accessed April 3, 2012.

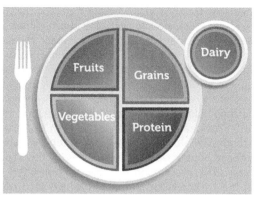

Fig. 1. Choose My Plate. (*From* United States Department of Agriculture. Choosemyplate. gov. Available at: http://www.choosemyplate.gov/index.html.)

Caution, Controversy, and Lack of Consensus

There are some points of concern and disagreement.

- *The DASH and TLC diets*[24,28]: These diets have recommended fruit servings of four to five 4-oz servings (DASH)[24] and four 4-oz servings (TLC),[25] respectively, of fruit or fruit juice, with several such servings allotted per day. A total of 20 oz (DASH) or 16 oz (TLC) of fruit juice could be consumed each day while still complying with guidelines. Dietary guidelines suggest whole fruit as better choices than fruit juice for those who are caries prone, diabetic, or obese because they provide more fiber and more satiety. Those choosing fruit juices instead of whole fruit on the DASH and TLC diet could be consuming 2 to 2.5

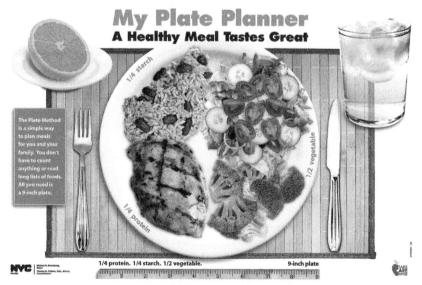

Fig. 2. My Plate Planner from the New York City, Department of Health. (*From* the New York City Department of Health and Mental Hygiene. Michael R. Bloomberg, Mayor Thomas R. Frieden, MD, MPH, Health Commissioner. Available at: http://www.nyc.gov/html/doh/downloads/pdf/csi/obesity-plate-planner-13.pdf.)

8-oz servings per day. Basch and coworkers[29] caution that not more than one fruit serving should be fruit juice and that juice quality differs in nutrient density. Constant between-meal sipping of juice is not one of the "five-a-day" recommendations. Using the Nurses' Health Study data, Bazzano and coworkers[30] discovered that with each increase of one serving per day of fruit juice (again defined as an 8-oz serving), the multivariate-adjusted relative risk of diabetes was 1.18.

- *De novo lipogenesis*: Frequent SSB consumption is thought to lead to high dietary glycemic load, inflammation, insulin resistance, and impaired pancreatic β-cell function.[31] Fructose from any sugar or high fructose corn syrup may promote the accumulation of visceral fat and ectopic hepatic fat deposition[11] because of increased hepatic de novo lipogenesis (de novo lipogenesis [DNL]).[32]
- *Uric acid pathway*: The association of SSBs and elevated blood pressure is consistent with the hypothesized effect of the uric acid pathway.[33] The uric acid pathway contributes to raised serum uric acid, which may influence blood pressure by reducing levels of nitric oxide, a potent vasodilator.[34] SSBs are the fourth most common source of calories in the United States and a clinician may find an immigrant adopting a Western diet with new complaints of abdominal/visceral fat, even in the absence of a change in weight. The clinician may see an increase in blood pressure over successive routine examinations. Asian populations are considered obese at lower body mass indexes than whites,[35] so initially, their risk may not be apparent to the clinician. Nakagawa and coworkers[34] provide a thorough review of the mechanisms underlying the physiologic changes leading to these elevations in blood pressure.
- *Human studies*: Human studies have pointed to differences in visceral fat accumulation when 25% of calories were provided with either glucose- or fructose-sweetened beverages. In 32 obese men visceral fat increased by 14% in the fructose-consuming group compared with about 5% in the control group, with no significant change in body weight or subcutaneous fat. De novo lipogenesis, a liver-mediated path of fructose metabolism, was increased and postprandial triglycerides increased, particularly at night.[32,36] In one small 10-week prospective study in humans, consuming either fructose or glucose, fasting plasma glucose and insulin levels increased and insulin sensitivity decreased in subjects consuming fructose, but not in those consuming glucose. The fructose consumption again increased DNL. Clinicians should be aware that visceral fat is metabolically active and intertwined in metabolic perturbance and metaflammation. Fructose is hypothesized to uniquely increase DNL, promote dyslipidemia, decrease insulin sensitivity, and increases visceral fat in adults who are overweight or obese.[32]
- *Satiety*: In some studies, very specific macronutrient choices contributed to weight gain or weight loss. Mozaffarian and colleagues[21] argue: "Strong positive associations with weight change were seen for starches, refined grains, and processed foods. These findings are consistent with results in limited short-term trials: consumption of starches and refined grains may be less satiating, increasing subsequent hunger signals, and total caloric intake, as compared with equivalent numbers of calories obtained from less processed, higher-fiber foods that also contain healthy fats and protein."[21,37]

Summary and Future Directions Regarding Nutrition and Oral Health

Historically, individual foods have not been linked to periodontal disease in the same manner that sugars act locally to affect caries.[7] However, periodontal disease management is bidirectional[38]: metabolic syndrome, obesity, and type 2 diabetes mellitus exacerbate periodontal disease severity,[39] and periodontal conditions contribute to and worsen systemic illness.[38,39] Taylor[38] and Susanto and coworkers[39] direct all clinicians to their crucial role in improving chronic disease biomarkers, such as blood pressure, fasting blood glucose, and triglycerides, through the aforementioned changes in nutrition. This is an urgently needed step toward mitigation of the pandemic of chronic debilitating disease across the globe. The next section describes promotion of physical activity to enhance primary and secondary prevention of disease.

GENERAL HEALTH BENEFITS OF PHYSICAL ACTIVITY

The general health benefits of physical activity in adults are well known[41] and include reduction in Coronary heart disease (CHD) risk[40,42]; reduced risk of depression,[43] stroke,[44] high blood pressure,[45] type 2 diabetes,[15] several cancers,[46] and improved bone density[47]; cognitive function[48]; and ability to maintain weight loss.[49] In children, many benefits are conferred, including but not limited to improved cardiorespiratory endurance and muscular fitness, bone health, favorable body composition, and reduced symptoms of anxiety and depression (**Box 1**).[50]

Physical Activity Recommendations

The consistency of the evidence, coupled with dose response, served as the basis for the most recent public health recommendations for physical activity in adults 18 to 65 years old,[51] and in children.[52] For older adults, a more detailed consideration about any specific impairment is required.[53] Current recommendations are for aerobic[51] and resistance[54] activities, to older adults[52] to those who have established diabetes[49] or CHD. General guidelines for children and adults were developed by the US Department of Health and Human Services, and published in a comprehensive report in 2008 (see **Box 2**).[50]

Summary of the Importance of Physical Activity

Currently, only a fraction of adults and children in the United States are physically active and the greatest benefits can be obtained by moving someone from the sedentary to a mild-moderately active level of activity. This is beneficial at all ages and it is never too early, or too late, to become physically active. As with dietary modification, the obstacles are considerable to successful change. Therefore, the next section addresses why change can be so difficult, and how the dentist can assist in the process of more successful change.

IMPROVING ORAL HEALTH OUTCOMES THROUGH PATIENT-CENTERED CARE

A major problem facing health professionals today is the lack of compliance with medical advice. Forty percent of all premature deaths in America are caused by poor health behaviors. These behaviors persist despite emphatic medical advice, warnings on cigarette packages, and legislation on nutrition labeling. In response to this reality, medical schools have implemented training in a variety of patient-centered approaches to the delivery of health information and health care. These include teaching awareness of health literacy levels of patients and the use of patient-centered care (PCC). PCC refines evidence-based guidelines to best address the individual's needs. Focus is placed on an empathic relationship and a collaborative spirit.

This section presents a rationale for the use of PCC in oral healthcare delivery to improve oral health outcomes.[55] Barriers to PCC from the patient's and practitioner's point of view are discussed. Included is a review of skills that can increase empathy and understanding, such as active listening and MI. This section is meant to familiarize

---

Box 1
Health benefits of physical activity: a review of the strength of the scientific evidence

ADULTS AND OLDER ADULTS

Strong Evidence

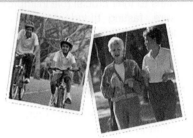

- Lower risk of
  - Early death
  - Heart disease
  - Stroke
  - Type 2 diabetes
  - High blood pressure
  - Adverse blood lipid profile
  - Metabolic syndrome
  - Colon and breast cancers
- Prevention of weight gain
- Weight loss when combined with diet
- Improved cardiorespiratory and muscular fitness
- Prevention of falls
- Reduced depression
- Better cognitive function (older adults)

Moderate to Strong Evidence

- Better functional health (older adults)
- Reduced abdominal obesity

Moderate Evidence

- Weight maintenance after weight loss
- Lower risk of hip fracture
- Increased bone density
- Improved sleep quality
- Lower risk of lung and endometrial cancers

CHILDREN AND ADOLESCENTS

Strong Evidence

- Improved cardiorespiratory endurance and muscular fitness
- Favorable body composition
- Improved bone health
- Improved cardiovascular and metabolic health biomarkers

Moderate Evidence

- Reduced symptoms of anxiety and depression[50]

Box 2
Key guidelines

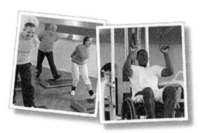

Substantial health benefits are gained by doing physical activity according to the Guidelines presented for different groups.

Children and Adolescents (aged 6–17)

- Children and adolescents should do 1 hour (60 minutes) or more of physical activity every day.
- Most of the 1 hour or more a day should be either moderate- or vigorous-intensity aerobic physical activity.
- As part of their daily physical activity, children and adolescents should do vigorous-intensity activity on at least 3 days per week. They also should do muscle-strengthening and bone-strengthening activity on at least 3 days per week.

Adults (aged 18–64)

- Adults should do 2 hours and 30 minutes a week of moderate-intensity, or 1 hour and 15 minutes (75 minutes) a week of vigorous-intensity aerobic physical activity, or an equivalent combination of moderate- and vigorous-intensity aerobic physical activity. Aerobic activity should be performed in episodes of at least 10 minutes, preferably spread throughout the week.
- Additional health benefits are provided by increasing to 5 hours (300 minutes) a week of moderate-intensity aerobic physical activity, or 2 hours and 30 minutes a week of vigorous-intensity physical activity, or a combination of both.
- Adults should also do muscle-strengthening activities that involve all major muscle groups performed on 2 or more days per week.

Older Adults (aged 65 and older)

- Older adults should follow the adult guidelines. If this is not possible because of limiting chronic conditions, older adults should be as physically active as their abilities allow. They should avoid inactivity. Older adults should do exercises that maintain or improve balance if they are at risk of falling.

For all individuals, some activity is better than none. Physical activity is safe for almost everyone, and the health benefits of physical activity far outweigh the risks. People without diagnosed chronic conditions (eg, diabetes, heart disease, or osteoarthritis) and who do not have symptoms (eg, chest pain or pressure, dizziness, or joint pain) do not need to consult with a healthcare provider about physical activity.

Adults with Disabilities

- Follow the adult guidelines. If this is not possible, these persons should be as physically active as their abilities allow. They should avoid inactivity.

Children and Adolescents with Disabilities

- Work with the child's healthcare provider to identify the types and amounts of physical activity appropriate for them. When possible, these children should meet the guidelines for children and adolescents—or as much activity as their condition allows. Children and adolescents should avoid being inactive.

Pregnant and Postpartum Women

- Healthy women who are not already doing vigorous-intensity physical activity should get at least 2 hours and 30 minutes (150 minutes) of moderate-intensity aerobic activity a week. Preferably, this activity should be spread throughout the week. Women who regularly engage in vigorous-intensity aerobic activity or high amounts of activity can continue their activity provided that their condition remains unchanged and they talk to their healthcare provider about their activity level throughout their pregnancy.[50]

readers with approaches to care that may improve compliance with lifestyle change. This is a cursory overview that requires additional exploration by the practitioner.

Compliance

Compliance with advice and treatment regimens in medicine is bleak. Nearly three out of four consumers admit to not taking prescription medications as directed.[56] Adherence rates for chronic illness rehabilitation regimens and lifestyle changes are approximately 50%.[57] It is difficult and frustrating for the health provider to meet with such resistance when attempting to help patients. Understanding the patient's perspective, perceived obstacles, and reasons for resistance may increase the possibility of a more collaborative approach.

Resistance to Change

There are complex reasons that patients do not follow health advice. This section addresses the issues of health literacy (patients not understanding advice), and mental health literacy (they have competing motivations for not changing).

Health literacy refers to "the degree to which individuals have the capacity to obtain, process, and understand basic health information and services needed to make appropriate health decisions."[58] It is a complex and multifaceted field, with many nuanced understandings of how people incorporate information.[59] The ADA specifically addresses the issue of oral health literacy and acknowledges the importance of health education and promotion in providing appropriate care to patients.[55] Clinicians can be sensitive to oral health literacy by simplifying the language they use to explain material, giving patients the opportunity to restate what they are being told, insure their understanding, and tailoring responses to their feedback.

Mental health literacy refers to awareness and appreciation of the patient's experience and capacity for change. Psychodynamics gives a framework to understand the motivations behind resistance or "noncompliance" of patients and one's own reactions as a health professional.

Issues for the Health Professional

In working with patients, the health professional brings training and skill, compassion and empathy, and a desire to help. However, he or she also brings judgments, defenses, and reactions to noncompliance. After all, professional identity depends on "success." Clinicians are disappointed in themselves and in their patients when they do not "get better." It is not surprising that medical students and residents become less empathic during training.[60] Ironically, training in the health professions can create obstacles in clinicians' efforts to help their patients. Whether it is because of fear of emotional involvement with people who are ill, the need to present oneself as an objective scientist, or frustration at the limitations of the healing professions, training can lead clinicians to create distance from patients and to treat them as people to be acted on.[61]

As clinicians begin to see patients' maladaptive behaviors as serving an underlying purpose and to understand their own reactions to these patients it becomes possible to replace judgments with understanding and frustration with empathy; clinicians can embark on an empathic collaborative relationship working together to improve health outcomes.

Patient-centered Care

Most healthcare providers are exposed to some information about PCC, and are aware of the need to regard patients as individuals. Usually the information is cursory and there is little emphasis placed on professional–patient interaction. Furthermore, there is little systematic teaching of specific tools to enhance collaborative relationships. PCC is not a panacea. It is an orientation that has shown some efficacy in promoting lifestyle changes and requires further research.[62] Two important and accessible tools for enhancing greater collaboration are active listening and MI.

Active Listening

Active listening is listening with focus and intent to give the other an opportunity to communicate thoughts, feelings, and concerns.[63] It is paying attention without interfering with the other's flow of information, and facilitating that flow. It includes asking open-ended questions reflecting, clarifying, summarizing, and most importantly sustaining a nonjudgmental stance. The techniques of active listening are detailed in **Box 3**.[63]

Motivational Interviewing

MI is a client-centered counseling approach geared specifically to patients' ambivalence in relation to behavior change. It is a methodology to resolve these ambivalences by empowering patients, respecting autonomy, and promoting self-efficacy. Often patients make comments, such as "I know I should refuse candy and desserts but I prefer to enjoy dessert when socializing with friends," and "I know I should floss but

---

Box 3
Active listening techniques

1. The use of body language: Showing interest through eye contact, body posture toward the patient. Paying attention to the patient's body language (eg, is he or she open or closed in body posture).

2. Asking open ended questions: It is important to show interest by asking patients to elaborate on what they are saying—to give them the stage to explore thoughts and feelings in your presence.

3. Reflecting clarifying and summarizing: Mirroring back (paraphrasing) what you heard gives the patient the knowledge that you are listening and when using phrases like "am I following you," gives the patient the opportunity to correct your understanding.

4. Sustaining a nonjudgmental stance: Practicing empathy allows us to put ourselves in our patients' shoes and understand the issue from their point of view. It means suspending our own point of view in the interests of understanding the other. It also means suspending advice giving.

It is through techniques such as these that patients will feel respected and understood. Such an attitude engenders a greater willingness to formulate and carry out behavior change.[63]

I already brush, and flossing is an added pain in the neck." These common statements provide an opportunity for the MI approach. The first step in MI is to determine the stage of change with the patient.[64] These stages include precontemplation (having no thoughts about the particular behavior); contemplation (considering the pros and cons of making a change); preparation (formulating a plan for change); action (implementing a plan); and maintenance (sustaining the change). At any point, relapse is possible. From the MI point of view, this is expected and planned for with the patient. It is not seen as failure, but part of the process of change.

At the stage of contemplation, advantages and disadvantages (from the patient's point of view) for the behavior are elicited. This is illustrated in the form of a matrix in **Box 4**[65] including the pros and cons of a patient changing, or not changing, a behavior when eating out with friends. Thus, ambivalence and issues of self-efficacy are explored through active listening and open-ended dialogue. This empowers patients to arrive at their own solutions with the support and guidance of a health professional.

Summary of the Role of the Practitioner in Assisting with Lifestyle Change

In the interests of providing the best possible health care, a method of improving patient/health practitioner communication has been explored. It is at the intersection between evidence-based care and the patient-centered approach that one hopes to bring about improved health behaviors. As is stated in the ADA Current Policies Document: "Patients need a dental home. All patients should have an ongoing relationship with a dentist with whom they can collaboratively determine preventive and restorative treatment appropriate to their needs and resources."[66] At the center of this collaborative effort is an opportunity for the dentist to offer nutrition and physical activity recommendations to prevent or mitigate chronic disease. This is an important expansion of the dentist's role in healthcare delivery.

CONCLUSIONS ON LIFESTYLE FACTORS AND ORAL HEALTH

Understanding the current dietary guidelines and physical activity recommendations is the first step to conveying key information to patients about the role of nutrition and activity in general and oral health. It is critical to move beyond classical views of the role of health providers, and to expand knowledge about the interaction of

Box 4 Patient's decision matrix		
	Eat Less Refined Carbohydrate Snacks and Sweets When Socializing	**Continue to Eat Refined Carbohydrate Snacks and Sweets When Socializing**
PROS	Help with weight loss Improve my insulin sensitivity Regulate blood sugar levels Improve oral health and reduce dental pain	Do not have to deal with peer pressure when refusing desserts Less anxiety about changing
CONS	Will have discomfort refusing dessert when dining with friends Will be anxious about changing Will feel insecure about meeting expectations	May gain more weight May not improve insulin sensitivity May feel less healthy Will not improve oral health, and will still have dental pain and expense

general health and oral health. This is seen most clearly in the interaction between diabetes and periodontal health, each potentially affecting the other in a downward spiral of worsening general health. Helping patients with proper weight management and physical activity are the challenges now and well into the future. Because the current nutrition and activity behaviors of most Americans is far from optimal, much can be gained as dentists develop a better understanding of the difficulties of sustained behavior change and become proficient in counseling approaches that lead to improved oral health for patients.

REFERENCES

1. Centers for Disease Control and Prevention Leading Causes of Death. Available at: http://www.cdc.gov/nchs/fastats/lcod.htm. Accessed April 2, 2012.
2. Shah K, Hunter ML, Fairchild RM, et al. A comparison of the nutritional knowledge of dental, dietetic and nutrition students. Br Dent J 2011;210(1):33–8.
3. Roger VL, Go AS, Lloyd-Jones DM, et al. Heart disease and stroke statistics—2012 update: a report from the American Heart Association. Circulation 2012;125(1):e2–220.
4. Yang Q, Cogswell ME, Flanders WD, et al. Trends in cardiovascular health metrics and associations with all-cause, and CVD mortality among US adults. JAMA 2012;307(12):1273–83.
5. Moynihan P, Petersen PE. Diet, nutrition and the prevention of dental diseases. Public Health Nutr 2004;7(1A):201–26.
6. Centers for Disease Control and Prevention. Achievements in public health, 1900–1999: fluoridation of drinking water to prevent dental caries. MMWR 1999;48:933–40.
7. Dye BA, Tan S, Smith V, et al. Trends in oral health status: United States, 1988–1994 and 1999–2004. National Center for Health Statistics. Vital Health Stat 11 2007;11(248):1–92.
8. Saint Louis C. Preschoolers in surgery for a mouthful of cavities. The New York Times 2012. Available at: http://www.nytimes.com/2012/03/06/health/rise-in-preschool-cavities-prompts-anesthesia-use.html?pagewanted=all. Accessed March 23, 2012.
9. U.S. Department of Agriculture and U.S. Department of Health and Human Services. Dietary guidelines for Americans. Washington, DC: U.S. Government Printing Office; 2010. Available at: http://www.health.gov/dietaryguidelines/2010.asp. Accessed April 1, 2012.
10. Ogden CL, Carroll MD, Kit BK, et al. Prevalence of obesity in the United States, 2009–2010. NCHS Data Brief 2012;82:1. Available at: http://www.cdc.gov/nchs/data/databriefs/db82.htm. Accessed March 30, 2012.
11. Bremer AA, Mietus-Snyder M, Lustig RH. Toward a unifying hypothesis of metabolic syndrome. Pediatrics 2012;129(3):557–70.
12. Gregor MF, Hotamisligil GS. Inflammatory mechanisms in obesity. Annu Rev Immunol 2011;29:415–45.
13. Serhan CN. Novel lipid mediators and resolution mechanisms in acute inflammation: to resolve or not? Am J Pathol 2010;177(4):1576–91.
14. Lloyd-Jones DM, Hong Y, Labarthe D, et al. Defining and setting national goals for cardiovascular health promotion and disease reduction: the American Heart Association's strategic impact goal through 2020 and beyond. Circulation 2010;121:586–613.
15. Knowler WC, Barrett-Connor E, Fowler SE, et al. Reduction in the incidence of type 2 diabetes with lifestyle intervention or metformin. N Engl J Med 2002;346(6):393–403.

16. Steinberger J, Daniels SR, Eckel RH, et al. Progress and challenges in metabolic syndrome in children and adolescents a scientific statement from the American Heart Association atherosclerosis, hypertension, and obesity in the young committee of the council on cardiovascular disease in the young; council on cardiovascular nursing; and council on nutrition, physical activity, and metabolism. Circulation 2009;119:628–47.

17. American Dental Association current policies: prevention and health education. Policy on Obesity. 2009:420 Available at: http://www.ada.org/currentpolicies.aspx. Accessed April 3, 2012.

18. American Dental Association Current Policies: Integration of oral health and disease prevention principles in health education curricula 1996:683. Available at: http://www.ada.org/currentpolicies.aspx. Accessed April 3, 2012.

19. Ludwig DS. Technology, diet, and the burden of chronic disease. JAMA 2011;305(13):1352–3.

20. Ludwig DS. Weight loss strategies for adolescents: a 14-year-old struggling to lose weight. JAMA 2012;307(5):498–508.

21. Mozaffarian D, Hao T, Rimm EB, et al. Changes in diet and lifestyle and long-term weight gain in women and men. N Engl J Med 2011;364:2392–404.

22. Willcox DC, Willcox BJ, Todoriki H, et al. The Okinawan diet: health implications of a low-calorie, nutrient-dense, antioxidant-rich dietary pattern low in glycemic load. J Am Coll Nutr 2009;28(Suppl):500S–16S.

23. Institute of Medicine of the National Academies. Food and nutrition board. Dietary reference intakes tables: the complete set. Available at: www.iom.edu/?id=21381. Accessed April 2, 2012.

24. United States Department of Health and Human Services, National Institutes of Health, National Heart Lung and Blood Institute. Publication No. 06–4082. Your guide to lowering your blood pressure with DASH. Available at: http://www.nhlbi.nih.gov/health/public/heart/hbp/dash/new_dash.pdf. Accessed March 30, 2012.

25. Centers for Disease Control and Prevention. Can lifestyle modifications using therapeutic lifestyle changes (TLC) reduce weight and the risk for chronic disease? Available at: www.cdc.gov/nutrition/downloads/R2P_life_change.pdf. Accessed April 3, 2012.

26. United States Department of Agriculture Choose My Plate.gov. Available at: http://www.choosemyplate.gov/. Accessed April 3, 2012.

27. New York City Department of Health My Plate Planner. Available at: http://www.nyc.gov/html/doh/html/csi/csi-obesity.shtml. Accessed April 3, 2012.

28. United States Department of Health and Human Services, National Institutes of Health, National Heart Lung and Blood Institute NIH Publication No. 06–5235. Your guide to lowering your cholesterol with dash. Available at: http://www.nhlbi.nih.gov/health/public/heart/chol/chol_tlc.htm. Accessed March 29, 2012.

29. Basch CE, Zybert P, Shea S. 5-A-DAY: dietary behavior and the fruit and vegetable intake of Latino children. Am J Public Health 1994;84(5):814–8.

30. Bazzano LA, Li TY, Joshipura KJ, et al. Intake of fruit, vegetables, and fruit juices and risk of diabetes in women. Diabetes Care 2008;31(7):1311–7.

31. Schulze MB, Liu S, Rimm EB, et al. Glycemic index, glycemic load, and dietary fiber intake and incidence of type 2 diabetes in younger and middle-aged women. Am J Clin Nutr 2004;80(2):348–56.

32. Stanhope KL, Schwarz JM, Keim NL, et al. Consuming fructose-sweetened, not glucose sweetened, beverages increases visceral adiposity and lipids and decreases insulin sensitivity in overweight/obese humans. J Clin Invest 2009;119:1322–34.

33. Brown IJ, Stamler J, Van Horn L, et al. Sugar-sweetened beverage, sugar intake of individuals, and their blood pressure: international study of macro/micronutrients and blood pressure. Hypertension 2011;57(4):695–701.
34. Nakagawa T, Hu H, Zharikov S, et al. A causal role for uric acid in fructose-induced metabolic syndrome. Am J Physiol Renal Physiol 2006;290:F625–31.
35. Wen CP, David Cheng TY, Tsai SP, et al. Are Asians at greater mortality risks for being overweight than caucasians? redefining obesity for Asians. Public Health Nutr 2009;12(4):497–506.
36. Bray GA. Fructose: pure, white, and deadly? fructose, by any other name, is a health hazard. J Diabetes Sci Technol 2010;4(4):1003–7.
37. Bornet FR, Jardy-Gennetier AE, Jacquet N, et al. Glycaemic response to foods: impact on satiety and long-term weight regulation. Appetite 2007;49:535–53.
38. Taylor GW. Bidirectional interrelationships between diabetes and periodontal disease: an epidemiologic perspective. Ann Periodontol 2001;6(1):99–112.
39. Susanto H, Nesse W, Dijkstra PU, et al. Periodontitis prevalence and severity in Indonesians with type 2 diabetes. J Periodontol 2011;82(4):550–7.
40. Blair SN, Kampert JB, Kohl HW III, et al. Influences of cardiorespiratory fitness and other precursors on cardiovascular disease and all-cause mortality in men and women. JAMA 1996;276:205–10.
41. Ford ES, Zhao G, Tsai J, et al. Low-risk lifestyle behaviors and all-cause mortality. Am J Public Health 2011;101:1922–9.
42. Berry JD, Dyer A, Cai X, et al. Lifetime risks of cardiovascular disease. N Engl J Med 2012;366:321–9.
43. Kruisdijk FR, Hendriksen IJ, Tak EC, et al. Effect of running therapy on depression (EFFORT-D). Design of a randomised controlled trial in adult patients [ISRCTN 1894]. BMC Public Health 2012;12:50.
44. Gordon NF, Gulanick M, Costa F, et al. Physical activity and exercise recommendations for stroke survivors: an American Heart Association scientific statement from the council on clinical cardiology, subcommittee on exercise, cardiac rehabilitation, and prevention; the council on cardiovascular nursing; the council on nutrition, physical activity, and metabolism; and the Stroke Council. Circulation 2004;109(16):2031–41.
45. Fagard RH. Exercise is good for your blood pressure: effects of endurance training and resistance training. Clin Exp Pharmacol Physiol 2006;33:853–6.
46. Eheman C, Henley SJ, Ballard-Barbash R, et al. Annual report to the nation on the status of cancer, 1975–2008, featuring cancers associated with excess weight and lack of sufficient physical activity. Cancer 2012. http://onlinelibrary.wiley.com/store/10.1002/cncr.27514/asset/27514_ftp.pdf?v=1&t=h5tilpyt&s=4d64fd45 37035b8a44b492f19a8b2c9ba3472bf9 [Epub ahead of print]. Accessed April 1, 2012.
47. Borer KT. Physical activity in the prevention and amelioration of osteoporosis in women: interaction of mechanical, hormonal and dietary factors. Sports Med 2005;35:779–830.
48. Wang HX, Xu W, Pei JJ. Leisure activities, cognition and dementia. Biochim Biophys Acta 2012;1822:482–91.
49. Praet DF, Van Loon L. Optimizing the therapeutic benefits of exercise in type 2 diabetes. J Appl Physiol 2007;103:1113–20.
50. The Physical Activity Guidelines for Americans At-A-Glance: a fact sheet for professionals. Reference to the 2008 physical activity guidelines for Americans U.S. Department of Health and Human Services. Available at: http://www.health.gov/paguidelines/factsheetprof.aspx. Accessed March 29, 2012.

51. Haskell WL, Lee IM, Pate RR, et al. American College of Sports Medicine; American Heart Association. Physical activity and public health: updated recommendation for adults from the American College of Sports Medicine and the American Heart Association. Circulation 2007;116:1081–93.

52. Centers for Disease Control and Prevention. Trends in leisure time physical inactivity by age, sex and race/ethnicity—United States, 1994–2004. MMWR 2005;54: 991–4.

53. Nelson ME, Rejeski WJ, Blair SN, et al. Physical activity and public health in older adults: recommendation from the American College of Sports Medicine and the American Heart Association. Circulation 2007;116:1094–105.

54. Williams MA, Haskell WL, Ades PA. American Heart Association council on clinical cardiology; American Heart Association council on nutrition, physical activity, and metabolism. Resistance exercise in individuals with and without cardiovascular disease: 2007 update: a scientific statement from the American Heart Association council on clinical cardiology and council on nutrition, physical activity, and metabolism. Circulation 2007;116:572–84.

55. American Dental Association Current Policies: patient safety and quality of care 2005:321. Available at: http://www.ada.org/currentpolicies.aspx. Accessed April 3, 2012.

56. Schroeder SA. We can do better: improving the health of the American people. N Engl J Med 2007;357:1221–8.

57. Haynes RB, Taylor DW, Sackett DL. Compliance in health care. Baltimore (MD): Johns Hopkins University Press; 1979.

58. Institute of Medicine. Innovations in health literacy: workshop summary. Washington, DC: National Academies Press; 2011. Available at: www.nap.edu. Accessed April 9, 2012.

59. Zarcadoolas C. The simplicity complex: exploring simplified health messages in a complex world. Health Promot Int 2010. http://dx.doi.org/10.1093/heaapro/daq075. Oxford University Press.

60. Hojat M, Mangione S, Nasca TJ, et al. An empirical study of decline in empathy in medical school. Med Educ 2004;38:934–41.

61. Shapiro J. Walking a mile in their patients' shoes: empathy and othering in medical students' education. Philos Ethics Humanit Med 2008;3(10). Available at: http://www.peh-med.com/content/3/1/10. Accessed April 9, 2012.

62. Cambridge Handbook of Psychology, Health and Medicine, 2007. Available at: http://ezproxy.cul.columbia.edu. Accessed April 3, 2012.

63. Hoppe MH. Active listening (electronic resource): improve your ability to listen and lead. Greensboro (NC): Center for Creative Leadership; 2006.

64. Prochaska J, diClemente C. The transtheoretical approach: crossing traditional boundaries of therapy. Homewood (IL): Dow Jones-Irwin; 1984.

65. Miller W, Rollnick S. Motivational Interviewing: preparing people for change. 2nd edition. New York: Guilford Press; 2002.

66. American Dental Association Current Policies: Universal Healthcare Reform 2008:433. Improving oral health in America. Patients need a dental home. Available at: http://www.ada.org/currentpolicies.aspx. Accessed April 3, 2012.

Screening for Infectious Diseases in the Dental Setting

David A. Reznik, DDS

KEYWORDS

- Human immunodeficiency virus • Hepatitis C virus • Rapid testing • Patient attitudes

KEY POINTS

- Human immunodeficiency virus (HIV) and hepatitis C virus (HCV) are 2 systemic infectious diseases that dental health care professionals can help identify with the goal of improving health outcomes, addressing health disparities, and improving the quality and quantity of life.
- By identifying suspect oral lesions, as is the case with HIV infection, or offering rapid screening tests in the dental setting for both HIV and HCV, the dental team can play an important role in linkage to confirmatory diagnosis and care.

HUMAN IMMUNODEFICIENCY VIRUS IN THE UNITED STATES

The Centers for Disease Control and Prevention (CDC) estimates that there are 1.2 million people living with human immunodeficiency virus (HIV) infection in the United States.[1] Latest estimations indicate that about 50,000 Americans become infected with HIV annually, and this number remained stable between 2006 and 2010.[2] Approximately 20% of those living with HIV infection are unaware of their status.[1–3] Even with advances in rapid HIV diagnostics and medical treatments to manage this disease, approximately 33% of persons diagnosed with HIV in 2008 developed acquired immune deficiency syndrome (AIDS) within 1 year of diagnosis.[4] In the United States alone, more than 16,000 people with AIDS were estimated to have died in 2008, and nearly 594,500 people have died since the epidemic began.[3]

African Americans and Hispanics/Latinos are the racial/ethnic groups most affected by HIV. African Americans represent approximately 14% of the United States population, but accounted for 44% of all new HIV infections in 2010.[5] Hispanic/Latinos represent approximately 16% of the total United States population, yet accounted for 20% of all new HIV infections in 2009 (**Fig. 1**). Overall, in 2009 African American men had the highest rate of new HIV infections (103.9 per 100,000), followed by Hispanic/Latino men (39.9 per 100,000), and African American women (39.7 per 100,000).[5]

Although the annual number of new HIV infections remained stable, there was an estimated 21% increase in HIV incidence for people aged 13 to 29 years, driven by a 34%

Grady Health System, Emory University School of Medicine, 341 Ponce de Leon Avenue, Atlanta, GA 30308, USA
E-mail addresses: Dreznik@HIVdent.org; dreznik@gmh.edu

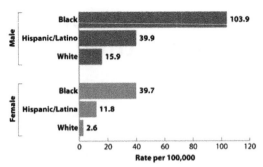

Fig. 1. Estimated rate of new HIV infections by gender and race/ethnicity, 2009. *Data from* Prejean J, Song R, Hernandez A, et al. (2011) Estimated HIV Incidence in the United States, 2006-2009. *PLoS ONE* 6(8):e17502. http://dx.doi.org/10.1371/journal.pone.0017502.

increase among young men who have sex with men (MSM).[3] CDC estimates MSM represent approximately 2% of the United States population, but accounted for more than 50% of all new HIV infections annually from 2006 to 2009 (**Fig. 2**).[5] Heterosexuals accounted for 27% (12,900) of estimated new HIV infections in 2009. There was no statistically significant change in HIV incidence overall among heterosexuals between 2006 and 2009.[6]

HEPATITIS C VIRUS IN THE UNITED STATES

Hepatitis C virus (HCV) infection is the most common blood-borne infection in the United States, with an estimated 3.2 million chronically infected persons.[7] Termed the silent epidemic, HCV is a leading cause of liver disease, cirrhosis, and death.[7] A total of 40 states and the District of Columbia submitted 781 reports of acute hepatitis C to the CDC in 2009.[8] When adjusted for underreporting, the number of acute hepatitis C cases decreased 78.4%, from 12,010 in 1992 to 2600 in 2009 (**Fig. 3**).[8] The incidence rate for 2009 was 0.3 cases per 100,000 population, and has remained unchanged since 2006.

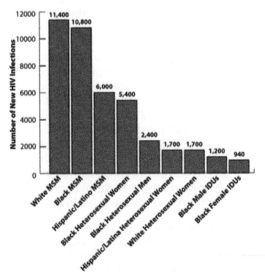

Fig. 2. Estimated new HIV infections by transmission category, 2009. *Data from* Prejean J, Song R, Hernandez A, et al. (2011) Estimated HIV Incidence in the United States, 2006-2009. *PLoS ONE* 6(8):e17502. http://dx.doi.org/10.1371/journal.pone.0017502.

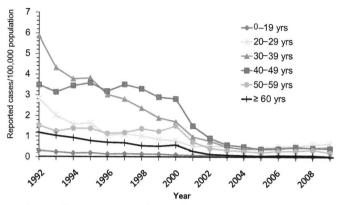

Fig. 3. Reported and adjusted number of acute hepatitis C cases in the United States, 1992 to 2009.

Persons newly infected with HCV are usually asymptomatic, so acute HCV is rarely identified or reported. Although surveillance infrastructure is in place for the reporting of acute infection, reports of chronic hepatitis B and C, which account for the greatest burden of disease, are not submitted by most states. As noted in a recent report from the Institute of Medicine, surveillance capacity to monitor both acute and chronic viral hepatitis is limited at the state and local levels, resulting in incomplete and variable data.[9]

Infection with HCV is most prevalent among the baby-boomer generation (those born during 1945 and 1965), the majority of whom were likely infected during the 1970s and 1980s.[10] The most common means of HCV transmission is via injection drug use (IDU).[10] Recent surveys of active injection-drug users (IDUs) indicate that approximately one-third of young IDUs (aged 18–30 years) are infected with HCV. Older and former IDUs typically have a much higher prevalence (approximately 70%–90%) of HCV infection, reflecting the increased risk of continued injection-drug use. The high HCV prevalence among former IDUs is largely attributable to nee-dle sharing during the 1970s and 1980s, before the risks of blood-borne viruses were widely known and before educational initiatives were implemented.[10] Others at risk for HCV infection include recipients of donated blood, blood products, and organs, considerably more common before blood screening became available in 1992; recip-ients of clotting-factor concentrates made before 1987; chronic hemodialysis pa-tients; those with needlestick injuries in health care settings; persons born from an HCV-infected mother; and persons living with HIV/AIDS.[10]

Since 2007, HCV has surpassed HIV as a cause of death in the United States.[11] Between 1999 and 2007, recorded deaths due to HCV increased to 15,106 and occurred disproportionately in middle-aged persons. During the same time period deaths from HIV declined to 12,734.[11] Factors associated with HCV deaths include chronic liver disease, minority status, hepatitis B virus coinfection, alcohol-related conditions, and HIV coinfection.[11] Achieving decreases in mortality, similar to those seen with HIV, will require new initiatives to detect patients with chronic disease and link them to appropriate care and treatment.

HIV SCREENING RECOMMENDATIONS

In 2006, the CDC updated the recommendations for HIV testing for health care providers in the public and private sectors. The revised guidelines called for one-time routine screening of all patients ages 13–64 years, repeated annually for high-risk groups. The rationale for the updated recommendations were due in part to the following factors: decreased effectiveness of risk-based screening; the failure to identify HIV infection even when patients access medical care; the low percentage of those that test positive in conventional settings returning for their results; and a failure to increase the number of people tested for HIV per year.[12]

Another important factor in updating the recommendations was to identify HIV-positive individuals earlier in the course of their disease. Early diagnosis of HIV can lead to a healthier and more productive life, improve the outcomes of early antiretroviral treatment, and is cost-effective over time.[13–15] In addition, early diagnosis may reduce HIV transmission rates because persons who know they are HIV-positive significantly reduce behaviors that would put others at risk.[16,17] Finally, results from the landmark HIV Prevention Trial Network 052 revealed that early initiation of antiretroviral therapy by HIV-infected individuals resulted in a 96% reduction in HIV transmission to their HIV-uninfected sexual partners.[18]

HCV TESTING RECOMMENDATIONS

HCV testing is recommended for routine screening of asymptomatic persons based on their risk of infection by recognized exposure.[19] The CDC currently recommends antibody screening of persons with past behaviors, exposures, or health indicators associated with HCV infection, such as a history of injection-drug use, hemodialysis, or elevated alanine aminotransferase (ALT) levels.[20] ALT is normally found in the liver; elevated ALT levels in the bloodstream signal liver disease or damage. However, 50% to 75% of people living with chronic HCV infection are unaware of their status.[21]

A recent publication suggests a cost-effective approach would be to screen the birth cohort born from 1945 through 1965, as a potential complement to current risk-based screening recommendations.[22] Compared with the present recommendations, birth-cohort screening would identify 808,570 cases, 95.9% of all undiagnosed cases in the birth cohort, compared with 21% under risk-based screening.[22] Without new HCV testing strategies, the impact of chronic HCV infection on public health in the next 2 decades will be significant. Deaths due to HCV are expected to double to more than 18,000 per year in 2020 and increase to 35,000 in 2030.[23]

HIV SCREENING IN THE DENTAL SETTING

In the early 1990s, oral manifestations of HIV were estimated to present at least once in 90% of people living with HIV/AIDS (PLWHA) and were often the first clinical signs of HIV disease.[24] More recent estimates have shown that the incidence of HIV-related oral lesions has markedly decreased since the advent of successful combination antiretroviral therapy.[25] At present, HIV-related oral conditions may occur at least once over the course of the disease in as few as 30% of PLWHA.[25,26] For individuals with unknown HIV status, certain oral manifestations such as pseudomembranous candidiasis may suggest HIV infection, although they are not diagnostic (**Fig. 4**).[27] Treatment of candidiasis by the dental practitioner followed by a referral to their primary care provider for a comprehensive workup, including HIV screening, is an appropriate course of action. If a dental practitioner notices an oral lesion such as Kaposi sarcoma, which is highly associated with HIV infection, it is appropriate to perform a biopsy and then schedule the patient with their primary care provider. A biopsy is necessary to confirm a diagnosis of Kaposi sarcoma before initiation of chemotherapy. If the patient does not have a primary care provider, referral to an infectious disease physician is strongly recommended. It should be noted, however, that risk-based screening or

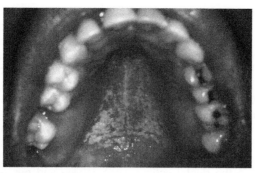

Fig. 4. Pseudomembranous candidiasis.

screening based on the presence of an oral lesion seen in association with HIV infection is not in agreement with the CDC's 2006 HIV testing recommendations. However, for the practitioner who does not want to offer HIV screening for all patients, identifying oral conditions seen in association with HIV disease followed by referral to a HIV testing facility or primary care provider will meet the intent of the US National AIDS Strategy.[28]

The National AIDS Strategy calls for an increase from 79% who presently know their HIV serostatus to 90% who are aware of their serostatus by 2015.[28] Data from the 2005 National Health Interview Survey revealed that 3.6 million Americans report that they are at significant HIV risk yet have never been tested.[29] Three-quarters of these individuals had seen a dental health care worker within the prior 2 years, and the investigators concluded that these dental visits represent missed opportunities to provide HIV testing for high-risk individuals.[29] Dental offices represent novel settings to reach millions in the United States who visit a dentist during the course of a year, but who do not see a physician,[30] and can serve as additional sites to identify health issues among diverse groups of patients.[30]

The US Food and Drug Administration has approved 6 rapid HIV antibody screening tests, 4 of which have obtained a Clinical Laboratory Improvement Amendments of 1988 (CLIA) waiver. CLIA specifies that laboratory requirements be based on the complexity of the test performed and establishes provisions for categorizing a test as waived. Waived tests are defined as laboratory examinations and procedures that are so simple and accurate as to render the likelihood of erroneous results negligible, or that pose no reasonable risk of harm to the patient if the test is performed incorrectly. Rapid HIV tests provide results in 20 minutes, eliminating the need for the patient to return at a later date, and account for an increased proportion of all HIV tests in the United States.[31] The advantages of rapid HIV tests, particularly with oral fluid specimens, include increased acceptability of testing among populations at risk as well as increased receipt of their test results.[32]

Studies have revealed a high patient acceptance rate when offered a free rapid HIV test in the dental setting.[33,34] In an attitude-assessment study piloted by the Kansas City Free Health Clinic at their stand-alone dental clinic located in a neighborhood with a high HIV prevalence, 73% of the 150 respondents were willing to take a free, oral fluid HIV screening test in the dental setting. Ninety-one percent of Hispanics, 79% of Caucasians, and 73% of African Americans were willing to be screened.[33] This study concluded that rapid HIV screening in the dental setting was a viable option to increase the number of people who would know their HIV status.[33] Once the Kansas City Free Clinic began to offer HIV screening to their dental patients, 6 newly diagnosed cases were found in an 18-month period out of 817 individuals tested.[35]

Harlem Hospital Center, located in New York City, instituted a counselor-based HIV screening initiative in their dental clinic.[34] As patients waited for their dental appointment, a trained counselor tested 3565 individuals, a 97.6% acceptance rate. Fifteen newly diagnosed individuals were linked to care, 6 of whom had a CD4 count of fewer than 200 cells/mm^3 and therefore by definition had AIDS at the time of their initial diagnosis. It was concluded that a counselor-based HIV screening program with linkage to HIV primary care can be successfully implemented in a large urban dental clinic.[34]

A study conducted at the New York University School of Dentistry, the largest provider of low-cost dental care in New York State, revealed that 74% of those approached would accept HIV screening if it were offered as a part of their dental visit.[36] This qualitative study revealed 3 themes regarding patients' views on rapid oral HIV screening in the dental setting: acceptability and perceived advantages; congruence between HIV screening and patients' view of dental settings and the roles of dental health care workers; and logistical issues related to implementation.[36] The identified logistical concerns included receiving preliminary reactive (positive) results, the need for professional counseling to address psychological concerns, and the importance of linkage to confirmatory testing and care.[36]

Linkage to confirmatory testing and care is integral to the success of HIV screening in the dental setting. Relationships should be in place with one of the following: a private practice infectious disease physician; a credentialed HIV medical provider; a state-funded disease intervention specialist; a Ryan White HIV/AIDS–funded program; a community health center with experience in managing HIV disease; a free health clinic with experience in managing HIV disease; or a linkage to an HIV care coordinator usually housed at an AIDS service organization. It is vitally important that these relationships be established during the planning phase of any initiative to screen patients for HIV disease. The Kansas City Free Health Clinic is a highly successful model that uses linkage-to-care case managers, who are paged by the dental staff when a preliminary reactive result is obtained and arrive at the dental facility within 20 minutes to manage the patient's follow-up, which includes confirmatory testing, risk-reduction counseling, and psychosocial support.[35]

The National Association of Community Health Centers (NACHC) in conjunction with the CDC has produced a toolkit for health centers that wish to initiate routine HIV screening in the dental setting.[37] This effort includes a comprehensive guide on all aspects of implementation, including words that dental health care professionals should consider using when offering this screening test. For example, stating that all patients aged 13 to 64 years are recommended to be screened at least once for HIV infection (annually for high-risk groups) and that the dental office is now offering this service to this age group as a part of routine care alleviates concerns about risk-based screening. "If you would like to receive a screening for HIV we will simply swab your gums. This oral swab tests for HIV antibodies, which are what your body produces if you are infected with HIV. The test gives results in twenty minutes (and is done while you are here for your visit). The results are accurate 99% of the time. Would you like to have an HIV oral test today?"[37] This effort also includes how to communicate nonreactive (negative) and reactive (positive) results. A nonreactive result indicates that the individual does not have antibodies to HIV. However, if the person believes they may have been infected in the past 3 months they should either be retested again in 3 months or be referred to an HIV testing center that has access to more specific diagnostic tests, such as a nucleic acid test. If the results are positive, NACHC's HIV toolkit recommends the following language. "Your oral swab showed that you may be infected with HIV. We call your results 'reactive' or 'preliminary' because we need to do more tests to know whether or not you are infected with

Table 1		
Resources for HIV screening in the dental setting		
HIV Screening Model for Dental Care	National Association of Community Health Centers	http://www.nachc.org/Dental%20Tools.cfm
HIV Testing in the Dental Chair: Technical Assistance Manual	New York/New Jersey AIDS Education and Training Center	http://www.nynjaetc.org/Testing.html
HIV Screening in the Dental Setting	HIV Dental Alliance (HIVDent)	http://www.hivdent.org/_hiv_screening/_hiv_screening_news.htm
Compendium of State HIV Testing Laws	National HIV/AIDS Clinicians Consultation Center	http://www.nccc.ucsf.edu/consultation_library/state_hiv_testing_laws/

HIV."[37] It is important to stress that HIV is now considered to be a chronic, manageable disease, no longer the death sentence it was in the earlier years of this epidemic. It is also important that a person with a preliminary reactive result be mindful that they need to protect themselves and others while they await a definitive diagnosis.

Finally, it is essential that a dental office undertaking this initiative follows state guidelines for HIV counseling and testing. The 2011 Compendium of State Testing Laws is a living document available through the National HIV/AIDS Clinicians Consultation Center housed at the University of California at San Francisco School of Medicine (**Table 1**).

HCV SCREENING IN THE DENTAL SETTING

Three rapid screening assays for HCV were submitted to the CDC for evaluation. The results revealed that a rapid anti-HCV test can provide sensitive and specific results for high-risk patients.[38] One rapid HCV antibody test, for which a CLIA waiver has been obtained, uses fingerstick whole blood or venous whole blood, and has a sensitivity of 97.8% to 99.3% with a specificity of 99.5%.[38] The CLIA waiver greatly increases the availability of this test in more than 180,000 facilities including outreach clinics, community-based organizations, and physician offices.[39]

Although rapid screening for HCV in the dental setting has not been investigated to date, the advances in medical management of this disease are occurring at a rapid rate. In 5 years, interferon-free direct-acting oral antiviral regimens may achieve close to 90% cure rates across viral genotypes.[40] A national "find and treat" initiative is required, aimed at identifying HCV-infected individuals and providing new-generation therapies for those infected.[40] Dental health care workers can play an important role in identifying cases of chronic HCV infection and linking these individuals into confirmatory testing and care.

SUMMARY

Dental health care workers provide an essential service by eliminating oral disease, promoting oral health, restoring function, and improving esthetics. Dental offices represent innovative settings reaching millions of individuals who visit a dentist during the course of a year, but who do not see a medical provider. This article highlights efforts that expand the role of the profession by screening for infectious diseases with the intent of reducing morbidity and mortality of the United States population. "It would be wrong to demand that all dental care providers perform HIV (HCV) tests in their offices. However, for the provider who will take the time to acquire the skills necessary to perform such a task, doing so could be a great benefit to society."[41]

REFERENCES

1. Centers for Disease Control and Prevention. HIV surveillance—United States, 1981-2008. MMWR Morb Mortal Wkly Rep 2011;60(21):689–93. Available at: http://www.cdc.gov/mmwr/PDF/wk/mm6021.pdf. Accessed March 1, 2012.
2. Prejean J, Song R, Hernandez A, et al. Estimated HIV Incidence in the United States, 2006-2009. PLoS One 2011;6(8):e17502.
3. Centers for Disease Control and Prevention. HIV in the United States. Available at: http://www.cdc.gov/hiv/resources/factsheets/us.htm. Accessed March 1, 2012.
4. Centers for Disease Control and Prevention. Vital signs: HIV testing and diagnosis among adults—United States, 2001-2009. MMWR Morb Mortal Wkly Rep 2010;59(47):1550–5.
5. Centers for Disease Control and Prevention. HIV/AIDS statistics and surveillance—HIV incidence. Available at: http://www.cdc.gov/hiv/topics/surveillance/incidence.htm. Accessed March 1, 2012.
6. Centers for Disease Control and Prevention. CDC Fact Sheet. Estimate of new HIV infections in the United States 2006-2009. 2011. Available at: http://www.cdc.gov/nchhstp/newsroom/docs/HIV-Infections-2006-2009.pdf. Accessed March 2, 2012.
7. Armstrong GL, Wasley AM, Simard EP, et al. The prevalence of hepatitis C virus infection in the United States, 1999 through 2002. Ann Intern Med 2006;144:705–14.
8. Centers for Disease Control and Prevention. Viral hepatitis surveillance—United States 2009. Available at: http://www.cdc.gov/hepatitis/Statistics/2009Surveillance/PDFs/2009HepSurveillanceRpt.pdf. Accessed March 3, 2012.
9. Institute of Medicine (IOM). Hepatitis and liver cancer: a national strategy for prevention and control of hepatitis B and C. Washington, DC: The National Academies Press; 2010.
10. Center for Disease Control and Prevention. Hepatitis C information for professionals. Available at: http://www.cdc.gov/hepatitis/HCV/index.htm. Accessed March 3, 2012.
11. Ly KN, Xing J, Klevens RM, et al. The increasing burden of mortality from viral hepatitis in the United States between 1999 and 2007. Ann Intern Med 2012;156:271–8.
12. Centers for Disease Control and Prevention. Revised recommendations for HIV testing of adults, adolescents, and pregnant women in health-care settings. MMWR Recomm Rep 2006;55(RR14):1–17. Available at: http://www.cdc.gov/mmwr/preview/mmwrhtml/rr5514a1.htm. Accessed March 3, 2012.
13. Hammer S, Eron J, Reiss P, et al. Antiretroviral treatment of adult HIV infection: 2008 recommendations of the International AIDS Society—USA Panel. JAMA 2008;300(5):555–70.
14. Walensky RP, Freedberg KA, Weinstein MC, et al. Cost-effectiveness of HIV testing and treatment in the United States. Clin Infect Dis 2007;45:S248–54.
15. Long EF, Brandeau ML, Owens DK. The cost-effectiveness and population outcomes of expanded HIV screening and antiretroviral treatment in the United States. Ann Intern Med 2010;153(12):778–89.
16. Marks G, Crepaz N, Senterfitt JW, et al. Meta-analysis of high-risk sexual behavior in persons aware and unaware they are infected with HIV in the United States: implications for HIV prevention programs. J Acquir Immune Defic Syndr 2005;39(4):446–53.

17. Marks G, Crepaz N, Janssen RS. Estimating sexual transmission of HIV from persons aware and unaware that they are infected with the virus in the USA. AIDS 2006;20(10):1447–50.
18. Cohen M, Ying C, McCauley M, et al. Prevention of HIV-1 Infection with early anti-retroviral therapy. N Engl J Med 2011;365:493–505.
19. Centers for Disease Control and Prevention. Sexually transmitted disease treatment guidelines, 2010. MMWR Recomm Rep 2010;59(RR12):1–110.
20. Recommendations for prevention and control of hepatitis C virus (HCV) infection and HCV-related chronic disease. Centers for Disease Control and Prevention. MMWR Recomm Rep 1998;47:1–39.
21. Wasley A, Finelli L, Bell B, et al. The knowledge and behaviors of HCV-infected persons identified in a seroprevalence survey, USA, 2001-2002. J Clin Virol 2006;36(Suppl 2):S198–9.
22. Rein D, Smith B, Wiitenborn BS, et al. The cost effectiveness of birth-cohort screening for Hepatitis C Antibody in U.S. Primary Care Settings. Ann Intern Med 2012;156:263–70.
23. Rein DB, Wittenborn JS, Weinbaum CM, et al. Forecasting the morbidity and mortality associated with prevalent cases of precirrhotic chronic hepatitis C in the United States. Dig Liver Dis 2011;43:66–72.
24. Weinert M, Grimes RM, Lynch DP. Oral manifestations of HIV infection. Ann Intern Med 1996;125:485–96.
25. Patton LL, McKraig R, Strauss R, et al. Changing prevalence of oral manifestations of human immunodeficiency virus in the era of protease inhibitor therapy. Oral Surg Oral Med Oral Pathol Oral Radiol Endod 2000;90:299–304.
26. Tani-Maury IM, Willig JH, Jolly PE, et al. Prevalence, incidence, and recurrence of oral lesions among HIV-infected patient on HAART in Alabama. South Med J 2011;104(8):561–6.
27. Reznik DA. Perspective—oral manifestations of HIV disease. Top HIV Med 2005–2006;13:143–8.
28. The White House Office of National AIDS Policy. National HIV/AIDS strategy for the United States. Washington, DC: White House; 2010.
29. Pollack HA, Metsch LR, Abel SA. Dental examinations as an untapped opportunity to provide HIV testing for high-risk individuals. Am J Public Health 2010; 100(1):88–9.
30. Strauss A, Alfano D, Shelley D, et al. Identifying unaddressed systemic health conditions at dental visits: patients who visited dental practices but not general health care providers in 2008. Am J Public Health 2012;102(2):253–5.
31. Association of Public Health Laboratories. Public Health Laboratory issues in brief: 2006 HIV diagnostic Survey. Silver Spring (MD): Association of Public Health Laboratories; 2007. Available at: http://www.aphl.org/aphlprograms/infectious/documents/hiv_issue_brief_2007.pdf. Accessed March 6, 2012.
32. Hutchinson AB, Branson BM, Kim A, et al. A meta-analysis of the effectiveness of alternative counseling and testing methods to increase knowledge of HIV status. AIDS 2006;20:1597–604.
33. Deitz CA, Ablah E, Reznik D, et al. Patient's attitudes about rapid oral HIV screening in an urban, free dental clinic. AIDS Patient Care STDS 2008;22(3):205–12.
34. Blackstok OJ, King JR, Mason RD, et al. Evaluation of rapid HIV testing initiative in an urban, hospital-based dental clinic. AIDS Patient Care STDS 2010;24(12):781–5.
35. Reznik DA, Neville S, Dietz CA, et al. Rapid oral HIV screening in the dental setting. Ryan White HIV/AIDS Program all grantees meeting. Washington, DC, 2008.

36. VanDevanter A, Combellick J, Hutchinson MK, et al. A qualitative study of patients' attitudes toward HIV testing in the dental setting. Nurs Res Pract 2012; 2012. Article ID 803169. http://dx.doi.org/10.1155/2012/803169.

37. HIV screening model for dental care. National Association of Community Health Centers. Last updated November 2010. Available at: http://www.nachc.org/Dental%20Tools.cfm. Accessed April 17, 2012.

38. Smith BD, Drobeniuc J, Jewett A, et al. Evaluation of three rapid screening assays for detection of antibodies to hepatitis C virus. J Infect Dis 2001;204(6):825–31.

39. Hepatology in focus. Gastroenterology and Endoscopy News, Hepatitis 2012;Vol 1.

40. Alter HJ, Liang TJ. Hepatitis C: the end of the beginning and possibly the beginning of the end. Ann Intern Med 2012;156(4):317–8.

41. Glick M. Rapid HIV testing in the dental setting. J Am Dent Assoc 2005;136:1208.

Assessment and Management of Patients with Diabetes Mellitus in the Dental Office

Evanthia Lalla, DDS, MS[a],*, Ira B. Lamster, DDS, MMSc[b]

KEYWORDS

- Diabetes • Oral health • Periodontitis • Management • Dentist • Primary care

KEY POINTS

- Dental professionals have the potential and the responsibility to assume an active role in the early identification, assessment, and management of their patients who present with or are at risk of developing diabetes.
- Periodontal prevention and intervention are imperative, but periodontal therapy may provide challenges. Close maintenance, meticulous monitoring of the individual patient needs at any given time, and close collaboration with other health care professionals involved in the patient's care will enable better control of the oral complications of diabetes and contribute to better management of the patient's overall health status.
- The time is right for implementing interprofessional education strategies in medical and dental training aiming to improve collaboration in the care of patients with diabetes.

DIABETES MELLITUS

Diabetes mellitus represents a group of common, chronic metabolic disorders characterized by abnormal glucose metabolism, caused by a defect in insulin secretion, insulin action, or both. Two major types of diabetes exist: type 1 and type 2. The latter type is far more prevalent, affecting 85% to 90% of the diabetic population.

Diabetes constitutes a serious public health concern worldwide; it requires lifelong care, leads to serious complications and premature death, and remains incurable. Globally, the number of adults with diabetes was estimated at 366 million for 2011 and is expected to rise to 552 million in 2030.[1] According to estimates in the United

---

The authors have nothing to disclose.
[a] Section of Oral and Diagnostic Sciences, Division of Periodontics, Columbia University College of Dental Medicine, 630 West 168th Street, PH7E-110, New York, NY 10032, USA; [b] Columbia University Mailman School of Public Health, Department of Health Policy & Management; Dean Emeritus, Columbia University College of Dental Medicine, 722 West 168th Street, New York, NY 10032, USA
* Corresponding author.
E-mail address: EL94@columbia.edu

States for 2010, diabetes mellitus affects 8.3% of its population (approximately 25.8 million people); among those 65 years of age and older, the prevalence is much higher (estimated at 26.9%).[2]

Hyperglycemia, the hallmark of both main types of diabetes, is associated with a range of acute and chronic disabling or life-threatening complications and can eventually affect all tissues and organs in the body, including the oral cavity. As a result, diabetes is relevant to all health care professionals, and the importance of prevention, early diagnosis, and proper treatment of affected individuals cannot be overstated.

ORAL COMPLICATIONS OF DIABETES MELLITUS
Periodontal Disease and the Two-Way Association

The effects of diabetes on the periodontal status of affected individuals have been extensively studied over many decades, and several reviews on the topic have been published.[3–5] In sum, among all systemic conditions, diabetes is the strongest risk factor for periodontitis, leading to increased prevalence, severity, and progression of the disease. Contrary to prior belief, diabetes can contribute to periodontal destruction even early in life, with recent comprehensive studies suggesting that diabetes significantly contributes to increased attachment loss in youth even after adjusting for common confounding factors.[6,7]

Importantly, the relationship of diabetes mellitus and periodontal disease seems to be bidirectional, with accumulating evidence suggesting that periodontal infections may adversely affect metabolic control and other health outcomes in patients with diabetes. Several longitudinal studies have shown that severe periodontitis at baseline, when compared with periodontal health or mild periodontitis, can lead to increased levels of hemoglobin A1c (HbA1c), increased mortality from cardiovascular outcomes, and more renal and vascular complications in patients with diabetes at follow-up.[8–11] Some evidence shows that severe periodontitis can also lead to incident diabetes,[12] although this concept has been challenged.[13] These effects are believed to be mediated through the proinflammatory mediators produced in the highly vascular periodontal tissue when periodontitis is present,[14,15] which can act as insulin antagonists.[16–18] Studies of periodontal treatment in patients with diabetes with systemic outcomes provide further support of these potential effects. Most of the available studies to date included small numbers of subjects and approached therapy with various protocols, but evidence from recent meta-analyses of treatment studies suggests that periodontal therapy will improve oral health for patients with diabetes, and this may also result in modest improvement in levels of metabolic control.[19,20]

Other Oral Complications

In addition to periodontal diseases, dental caries, burning mouth syndrome, *Candida* infection, salivary dysfunction/xerostomia, taste and other neurosensory disorders, altered tooth eruption and benign parotid hypertrophy have all been reported to be associated with diabetes.[21]

Evidence suggests that tooth eruption in the late mixed dentition period is accelerated in youth with diabetes compared with those without.[22] On the other end of the age spectrum, some of the more recent findings in older adults include the following: (1) coronal caries seem comparable, but the prevalence of root caries is higher in patients with diabetes[23]; (2) salivary flow is comparable, but the effects of xerogenic medications are more pronounced in patients with diabetes than controls[24]; and (3) for edentulous patients with diabetes, a greater prevalence of burning mouth syndrome, dry mouth, angular cheilitis, and glossitis is observed.[25]

These disorders have received less attention than periodontitis in the literature, but given the increasing prevalence of diabetes in both children and older adults and the aging of the population, several patients may present with a diabetes-related oral complaint and, thus, awareness of these potential oral disorders in patients with diabetes is important for dental practitioners.

PATIENT AND HEALTH CARE PROVIDER AWARENESS OF THE LINK BETWEEN DIABETES AND ORAL HEALTH

The variety of oral complications associated with diabetes emphasizes their importance for patients and the medical and dental professionals who care for them. Still, studies suggest relatively low awareness of these issues among patients and professionals alike.

According to Tomar and Lester,[26] patients with diabetes were less likely to visit a dentist in the preceding 12 months, and the leading reason for not seeing a dentist was "lack of perceived need." Moore and colleagues[27] also reported that only 18% of patients with diabetes were aware of its effects on oral health and 52% reported cost as the reason for avoiding routine dental visits. Subsequent studies in the United-States,[28–30] Sweden,[31,32] the United Kingdom,[28] and Jordan[33] suggested similar trends.

With regard to medical providers, the evidence to date suggests that physicians and nurses do not receive adequate training in oral health, rarely advise patients on aspects of oral health, and are not comfortable performing a simple periodontal examination on their at-risk patients.[34–37] A more recent survey of North Carolina endocrinologists and internists (response rate: 34%) showed that physicians believe an association exists between periodontitis and diabetes.[38] However, most are not aware of the studies that link the conditions and believe that physicians should receive more education about periodontal diseases and how to screen for them.

Dental professionals are largely aware of the link between diabetes and oral health, because related material has been taught in dental and dental hygiene schools for many decades, but unfortunately this knowledge does not seem to fully translate into practice. Some years ago, dentists' performance of activities related to the management of patients with diabetes was investigated via a mail survey of a representative sample of randomly selected general practitioners and periodontists in the northeast United States (response rate: 80% and 73%, respectively).[39–41] Results showed that general dentists are more willing to manage the care of patients with diabetes on an assessing and advising basis than on a more active management basis. With respect to periodontists, results were similar, although overall periodontists performed active management behaviors more frequently than general dentists. When assessed internationally in a representative sample of general dentists in New Zealand, a similar pattern of involvement emerged.[42] Since these first reports documenting the extent of dentists' practice activities with respect to the management of patients with diabetes, and with increasing evidence of the oral-systemic link, subsequent studies have suggested that attitudes toward active management have somewhat improved.[43,44]

ASSESSMENT AND MANAGEMENT OF PATIENTS WITH DIABETES MELLITUS BY DENTAL PROFESSIONALS

The information reviewed earlier strongly suggests a great need, and responsibility, for dental professionals to assume an active role in the education and management of patients with diabetes. Encouragingly, several characteristics of dental practice are consistent with dentists assuming this role: they treat large numbers of patients each year, and often provide primary and preventive care that is nonemergent in nature. Even patients who attend dental offices for "problem-oriented" visits often segue into preventive programs and regular examination and hygiene visits after completion of active treatment, and are seen at regular recall intervals. This practice allows for certain conditions to be followed over time and provides an opportunity for long-term patient contact and reinforcement.

Diagnosis and treatment of diabetes mellitus are the responsibility of the physician. However, as outlined in **Box 1**, dental professionals have a responsibility to seek to identify patients at risk who may remain uninformed and undiagnosed; evaluate signs and symptoms indicative of poor metabolic control in patients with known diabetes; advise identified patients in both groups about their condition and refer them to a physician for proper evaluation and treatment; and provide safe and predictable oral care for all of these patients, as needed.

Patient with Unknown Diabetes or at Risk for Developing Diabetes

Currently, an estimated one-quarter of patients affected by diabetes in the United States remain undiagnosed.[2] Because symptoms in type 2 diabetes develop gradually and are not specific to the disease, the diagnosis is frequently not made until complications appear.[45] The delay in clinical diagnosis is substantial and involves a period of about 9 to 12 years.[46] Type 1 diabetes is considered not preventable, but type 2 diabetes can be prevented in many cases, and awareness of its major risk factors (outlined in **Box 2**), many of which are modifiable, is important. Further, prediabetes (a condition in which blood glucose levels are higher than normal, but not high enough for a diagnosis of diabetes) affects approximately 35% of the U.S. adult population.[2] People with prediabetes have a strong risk for developing type 2 diabetes and are already at an increased risk for heart disease, stroke, and microvascular diseases.[47] Strong evidence indicates that people with prediabetes who lose weight and increase their physical activity can prevent or delay diabetes and even return their blood glucose levels to normal.[48] As with diabetes, the paramount challenge is early detection and intervention, and all health care providers can contribute to improved patient awareness and appropriate patient management.

Early identification of people with, or at risk for, diabetes can clearly not be the sole responsibility of the medical community or any single group of health care providers. The discovery of additional numbers of patients unaware of their prediabetic or diabetic state can have significant health care implications, especially in high-risk minority communities, because diabetes is more prevalent in immigrants, communities with

---

Box 1
Responsibilities of dental professionals toward patients at risk for, or with known, diabetes mellitus

- Know the major type 2 diabetes risk factors and seek to identify dental patients at risk who may remain unidentified/undiagnosed
- Evaluate signs and symptoms indicative of poor metabolic control in patients with known diabetes
- Inform identified patients in both groups about their condition and advise on lifestyle modifications
- Refer patients in both groups to a physician for proper evaluation and treatment
- Provide safe and predictable oral/dental care, as needed

Box 2
Risk factors for type 2 diabetes mellitus

- Age >40 years (or younger for high-risk race/ethnicity individuals)
- High-risk race/ethnicity (African American, Hispanic/Latino, Alaska Native, American Indian, Asian American, or Pacific Islander)
- Family history of diabetes (1st- or 2nd-degree relative)
- Habitual physical inactivity
- Overweight (body mass index $\geq$25 kg/m^2 for most but not all ethnic groups)
- Hypertension (blood pressure $\geq$140/90 mm Hg)
- Dyslipidemia (high-density lipoprotein cholesterol $\leq$35 mg/dL or triglycerides $\geq$250 mg/dL)
- Prediabetes, impaired glucose tolerance, or impaired fasting glucose
- History of vascular disease or other diabetes-associated conditions
- For women
  - Delivery of infant >9 lb
  - History of gestational diabetes
  - Polycystic ovary syndrome

---

lower socioeconomic status, and minorities.[2,49–53] The American Diabetes Association Standards of Medical Care[54] suggest that diabetes testing should be only performed within a health care setting, because of the need for follow-up. Community screening is not recommended because people with positive tests may not have access to appropriate follow-up, those with negative tests may not be able to be reached or undergo appropriate repeat testing, those at high risk may not be able to be reached, or inappropriate testing may be performed in those at low risk.

Combining risk factors, easily identifiable during a patient's routine medical history-taking, with oral findings in affected individuals who remain undiagnosed can be a valuable strategy in a dental setting. With this concept in mind, a national sample of 4830 U.S. adults from the National Health and Nutrition Examination Survey (NHANES) III public-use files were analyzed and probabilities of undiagnosed diabetes using periodontal parameters as part of the equation were calculated.[55] The analyses revealed that individuals with 3 self-reported risk factors (family history of diabetes, hypertension, high cholesterol levels) and clinical evidence of periodontal disease bear a probability of 27% to 53% of having undiagnosed diabetes, with Mexican American men exhibiting the highest probability and white women the lowest. These data suggested that such a simple approach offers an unrealized opportunity to identify individuals affected by diabetes who remain unaware of their condition in dental settings. This notion was supported by data from similar approaches in 2 subsequent NHANES-based studies.[56,57]

These concepts were then tested for the first time prospectively in a dental clinic population, and potentially unrecognized prediabetes was included in the equation. A first report in 2011[58] analyzed data from 506 new, at-risk dental patients and provided evidence that the presence of at least 26% of teeth with at least one deep pocket ($\geq$5 mm) or at least 4 missing teeth can correctly identify 73% of true cases of previously unrecognized diabetes or prediabetes. The addition of a point-of-care HbA1c result of 5.7% or more increased correct identification to 92%. When optimal cutoffs were used, performance characteristics of the 2-dental-variable model were similar to those of a point-of-care HbA1c alone. The 2 identified predictive models have high sensitivity, similar to what has been reported for diabetes risk assessment approaches tested in medical settings.[59] False-positive results are less significant in this context, because the dental professional will not make or deliver a formal diagnosis to the patient. The dentist's role would be to (1) alert identified patients that they are at high risk for or may actually have diabetes, (2) advise them on healthy lifestyle changes and modifiable risk factors, (3) direct them to seek further testing and advice from a physician and, importantly, (4) follow-up on the outcome at future dental visits.

Subsequently, other investigators supported the notion of screening for undiagnosed diabetes in dental settings and provided evidence that implementation of diabetes testing in dental practices is feasible, and that both patients and dental providers believe that the dental visit is a good opportunity for early diabetes identification.[60,61]

Patient with Known Diabetes

Similarly to primary prevention, secondary and tertiary prevention in diabetes are of essence. Unfortunately, evidence shows that achieving treatment goals remains challenging for a large number of patients with diabetes.[62]

To support people with diabetes in their effort to achieve better outcomes and avoid or delay the development of complications, the importance of good glycemic control and a healthy lifestyle must be reviewed and emphasized at every contact with the health care system, including any dental visits. Dental practitioners must join other health care professionals in providing their patients with diabetes with guidance in goal setting, suggesting strategies on how to achieve goals and techniques to overcome barriers, providing self-management training, and screening and managing the risk for complications. They also need to provide continuous patient reinforcement and support. In terms of oral health education, dental professionals must discuss with their patients the link between oral and general health, how diabetes and periodontitis interrelate, and the need for comanagement of their condition by multiple health care providers. They must promote lifestyle changes and good oral health behaviors.

Additionally, dental professionals can help increase awareness about the association between diabetes and oral health among their colleagues in medicine and promote activities among medical care providers that can lead to better health outcomes in common patients. These activities in medical settings include (1) discussing the importance of oral health and its relationship to diabetes, and the potential sequelae of longstanding, untreated oral infections; (2) advising patients with poorly controlled diabetes to see a dentist on a regular basis; (3) immediate referral to a dentist for patients with diabetes who report that they have not seen a dentist in the past year, or those who have seen a dentist in the past year but present with detectable signs or symptoms of oral infections; (4) screening for oral/periodontal changes, similar to screening for other complications, through asking about symptoms and/or performing a simple visual assessment of the mouth; and (5) facilitating communication with the treating dentist through offering information on patients' medical background and being available to offer advice on medical management modifications that may be necessary.

Dental professionals must also ensure that the oral care they deliver to their patients with diabetes is safe, and that therapeutic outcomes are predictable. To this end, some special considerations in the dental treatment of patients with diabetes include taking a thorough medical history and establishing communication with the treating physician. A careful intraoral evaluation is key (**Box 3**) and should include a complete

---

Box 3
Components of a thorough oral evaluation in patients with known diabetes mellitus

- Whole-mouth periodontal evaluation consisting of
  - Probing depth and attachment loss measurements
  - Assessment of the level of plaque and gingival inflammation
  - Radiographic evaluation of bone levels, as needed
- Thorough examination for oral mucosal lesions (eg, lichen planus, apthous stomatitis)
- Identification of signs and symptoms of opportunistic infections (eg, oral candidiasis)
- Evaluation of salivary flow
- Assessment of taste disturbances and signs/symptoms of burning mouth syndrome
- Crown and root caries assessment

---

periodontal evaluation with whole-mouth probing depth and attachment loss measurements, assessment of plaque and gingival inflammation, and radiographic evaluation of bone levels as needed; a thorough examination for oral mucosal lesions (eg, lichen planus, apthous stomatitis); identification of signs and/or symptoms of opportunistic infections (eg, oral candidiasis); evaluation of salivary flow; assessment of taste disturbances and signs/symptoms of burning mouth syndrome; and dental caries assessment. Initial therapy should focus on the control of any acute infections identified and a less complex stepwise therapy plan should be promoted when possible.

Finally, prevention, early recognition, and proper management of emergencies in the dental office are also very important. Dental professionals must remember that hypoglycemic episodes are common in all people with type 1 and many with advanced type 2 diabetes. Hyperglycemic crisis is less common but serious. Dental professionals must therefore consider timing and duration of appointments and the possible need for change in diabetic regimen in consultation with the treating physician. They must provide profound anesthesia and pain control in conjunction with invasive procedures, along with any antibiotic, anti-inflammatory, or host modulation agents. Clinical protocols and guidelines should be in place in every dental practice setting for determining frequency of follow-up care, the need for referral to a dental specialist ,and the need for medical consultation, referral, and follow-up.

SUMMARY

Diabetes mellitus is a serious chronic disease that affects many dental patients. Dental professionals have the potential and responsibility to assume an active role in the early identification, assessment, and management of their patients who present with or are at risk of developing diabetes. Periodontal prevention and intervention are imperative, but periodontal therapy may provide challenges. Close maintenance, meticulous monitoring of the individual patient needs at any given time, and close collaboration with other health care professionals involved in the care of the patient will allow for better control of the oral complications of diabetes and will contribute to the better management of the patient's overall health status. The time is right for implementing interprofessional education strategies in medical and dental training aiming to improve physicians' and dentists' collaboration in the care of patients with diabetes.

REFERENCES

1. IDF Diabetes Atlas, Fifth Edition. The global burden: prevalence and projections. International Diabetes Federation Web site. Available at: http://www.idf.org/diabetesatlas/5e/the-global-burden. Accessed April 19, 2012.
2. Centers for Disease Control and Prevention. National diabetes fact sheet: national estimates and general information on diabetes and prediabetes in the United States, 2010. Atlanta (GA): U.S. Department of Health and Human Services, Centers for Disease Control and Prevention; 2011.
3. Mealey BL, Rose LF. Diabetes mellitus and inflammatory periodontal diseases. Curr Opin Endocrinol Diabetes Obes 2008;15(2):135–41.
4. Taylor GW, Borgnakke WS. Periodontal disease: associations with diabetes, glycemic control and complications. Oral Dis 2008;14(3):191–203.
5. Lalla E, Papapanou PN. Diabetes mellitus and periodontitis: a tale of two common interrelated diseases. Nat Rev Endocrinol 2011;7(12):738–48.
6. Lalla E, Cheng B, Lal S, et al. Periodontal changes in children and adolescents with diabetes: a case-control study. Diabetes Care 2006;29(2):295–9.
7. Lalla E, Cheng B, Lal S, et al. Diabetes mellitus promotes periodontal destruction in children. J Clin Periodontol 2007;34(4):294–8.
8. Taylor GW, Burt BA, Becker MP, et al. Severe periodontitis and risk for poor glycemic control in patients with non-insulin-dependent diabetes mellitus. J Periodontol 1996;67(Suppl 10):1085–93.
9. Thorstensson H, Kuylenstierna J, Hugoson A. Medical status and complications in relation to periodontal disease experience in insulin-dependent diabetics. J Clin Periodontol 1996;23(3 Pt 1):194–202.
10. Saremi A, Nelson RG, Tulloch-Reid M, et al. Periodontal disease and mortality in type 2 diabetes. Diabetes Care 2005;28(1):27–32.
11. Shultis WA, Weil EJ, Looker HC, et al. Effect of periodontitis on overt nephropathy and end-stage renal disease in type 2 diabetes. Diabetes Care 2007;30(2):306–11.
12. Demmer RT, Jacobs DR Jr, Desvarieux M. Periodontal disease and incident type 2 diabetes: results from the First National Health and Nutrition Examination Survey and its epidemiologic follow-up study. Diabetes Care 2008;31(7):1373–9.
13. Ide R, Hoshuyama T, Wilson D, et al. Periodontal disease and incident diabetes: a seven-year study. J Dent Res 2011;90(1):41–6.
14. Kebschull M, Demmer RT, Papapanou PN. "Gum bug, leave my heart alone!"–epidemiologic and mechanistic evidence linking periodontal infections and atherosclerosis. J Dent Res 2010;89(9):879–902.
15. Loos BG. Systemic markers of inflammation in periodontitis. J Periodontol 2005; 76(Suppl 11):2106–15.
16. King GL. The role of inflammatory cytokines in diabetes and its complications. J Periodontol 2008;79(Suppl 8):1527–34.
17. Shoelson SE, Lee J, Goldfine AB. Inflammation and insulin resistance. J Clin Invest 2006;116(7):1793–801.
18. Pradhan AD, Manson JE, Rifai N, et al. C-reactive protein, interleukin 6, and risk of developing type 2 diabetes mellitus. JAMA 2001;286(3):327–34.
19. Teeuw WJ, Gerdes VE, Loos BG. Effect of periodontal treatment on glycemic control of diabetic patients: a systematic review and meta-analysis. Diabetes Care 2010;33(2):421–7.

20. Simpson TC, Needleman I, Wild SH, et al. Treatment of periodontal disease for glycaemic control in people with diabetes. Cochrane Database Syst Rev 2010;(5):CD004714.
21. Lamster IB, Lalla E, Borgnakke WS, et al. The relationship between oral health and diabetes mellitus. J Am Dent Assoc 2008;139(Suppl):19S–24S.
22. Lal S, Cheng B, Kaplan S, et al. Accelerated tooth eruption in children with diabetes mellitus. Pediatrics 2008;121(5):e1139–43.
23. Meurman JH, Collin HL, Niskanen L, et al. Saliva in non-insulin-dependent diabetic patients and control subjects: the role of the autonomic nervous system. Oral Surg Oral Med Oral Pathol Oral Radiol Endod 1998;86(1):69–76.
24. Touger-Decker R, Mobley CC. Position of the American Dietetic Association: oral health and nutrition. J Am Diet Assoc 2003;103(5):615–25.
25. Dorocka-Bobkowska B, Zozulinska-Ziolkiewicz D, Wierusz-Wysocka B, et al. Candida-associated denture stomatitis in type 2 diabetes mellitus. Diabetes Res Clin Pract 2010;90(1):81–6.
26. Tomar SL, Lester A. Dental and other health care visits among U.S. adults with diabetes. Diabetes Care 2000;23(10):1505–10.
27. Moore PA, Orchard T, Guggenheimer J, et al. Diabetes and oral health promotion: a survey of disease prevention behaviors. J Am Dent Assoc 2000;131(9): 1333–41.
28. Allen EM, Ziada HM, O'Halloran D, et al. Attitudes, awareness and oral health-related quality of life in patients with diabetes. J Oral Rehabil 2008;35(3):218–23.
29. Yuen HK, Wolf BJ, Bandyopadhyay D, et al. Oral health knowledge and behavior among adults with diabetes. Diabetes Res Clin Pract 2009;86(3):239–46.
30. Moffet HH, Schillinger D, Weintraub JA, et al. Social disparities in dental insurance and annual dental visits among medically insured patients with diabetes: the Diabetes Study of Northern California (DISTANCE) Survey. Prev Chronic Dis 2010;7(3):A57.
31. Sandberg GE, Sundberg HE, Wikblad KF. A controlled study of oral self-care and self-perceived oral health in type 2 diabetic patients. Acta Odontol Scand 2001; 59(1):28–33.
32. Jansson H, Lindholm E, Lindh C, et al. Type 2 diabetes and risk for periodontal disease: a role for dental health awareness. J Clin Periodontol 2006;33(6): 408–14.
33. Al Habashneh R, Khader Y, Hammad MM, et al. Knowledge and awareness about diabetes and periodontal health among Jordanians. J Diabet Complications 2010;24(6):409–14.
34. Quijano A, Shah AJ, Schwarcz AI, et al. Knowledge and orientations of internal medicine trainees toward periodontal disease. J Periodontol 2010;81(3):359–63.
35. Al-Habashneh R, Barghout N, Humbert L, et al. Diabetes and oral health: doctors' knowledge, perception and practices. J Eval Clin Pract 2010;16(5):976–80.
36. Ward AS, Cobb CM, Kelly PJ, et al. Application of the theory of planned behavior to nurse practitioners' understanding of the periodontal disease-systemic link. J Periodontol 2010;81(12):1805–13.
37. Al-Khabbaz AK, Al-Shammari KF, Al-Saleh NA. Knowledge about the association between periodontal diseases and diabetes mellitus: contrasting dentists and physicians. J Periodontol 2011;82(3):360–6.
38. Owens JB, Wilder RS, Southerland JH, et al. North Carolina internists' and endocrinologists' knowledge, opinions, and behaviors regarding periodontal disease and diabetes: need and opportunity for interprofessional education. J Dent Educ 2011;75(3):329–38.

39. Kunzel C, Lalla E, Albert DA, et al. On the primary care frontlines: the role of the general practitioner in smoking-cessation activities and diabetes management. J Am Dent Assoc 2005;136(8):1144–53 [quiz: 1167].

40. Kunzel C, Lalla E, Lamster I. Dentists' management of the diabetic patient: contrasting generalists and specialists. Am J Public Health 2007;97(4):725–30.

41. Kunzel C, Lalla E, Lamster IB. Management of the patient who smokes and the diabetic patient in the dental office. J Periodontol 2006;77(3):331–40.

42. Forbes K, Thomson WM, Kunzel C, et al. Management of patients with diabetes by general dentists in New Zealand. J Periodontol 2008;79(8):1401–8.

43. Esmeili T, Ellison J, Walsh MM. Dentists' attitudes and practices related to diabetes in the dental setting. J Public Health Dent 2010;70(2):108–14.

44. Greenberg BL, Glick M, Frantsve-Hawley J, et al. Dentists' attitudes toward chairside screening for medical conditions. J Am Dent Assoc 2010;141(1):52–62.

45. Harris MI, Eastman RC. Early detection of undiagnosed diabetes mellitus: a US perspective. Diabetes Metab Res Rev 2000;16(4):230–6.

46. Harris MI, Klein R, Welborn TA, et al. Onset of NIDDM occurs at least 4-7 yr before clinical diagnosis. Diabetes Care 1992;15(7):815–9.

47. Diabetes Prevention Program Research Group. The prevalence of retinopathy in impaired glucose tolerance and recent-onset diabetes in the Diabetes Prevention Program. Diabet Med 2007;24(2):137–44.

48. Knowler WC, Barrett-Connor E, Fowler SE, et al. Reduction in the incidence of type 2 diabetes with lifestyle intervention or metformin. N Engl J Med 2002;346(6):393–403.

49. Riste L, Khan F, Cruickshank K. High prevalence of type 2 diabetes in all ethnic groups, including Europeans, in a British inner city: relative poverty, history, inactivity, or 21st century Europe? Diabetes Care 2001;24(8):1377–83.

50. Robbins JM, Vaccarino V, Zhang H, et al. Socioeconomic status and type 2 diabetes in African American and non-Hispanic white women and men: evidence from the Third National Health and Nutrition Examination Survey. Am J Public Health 2001;91(1):76–83.

51. Tucker KL, Bermudez OI, Castaneda C. Type 2 diabetes is prevalent and poorly controlled among Hispanic elders of Caribbean origin. Am J Public Health 2000; 90(8):1288–93.

52. Robbins JM, Vaccarino V, Zhang H, et al. Excess type 2 diabetes in African-American women and men aged 40-74 and socioeconomic status: evidence from the Third National Health and Nutrition Examination Survey. J Epidemiol Community Health 2000;54(11):839–45.

53. Brancati FL, Kao WH, Folsom AR, et al. Incident type 2 diabetes mellitus in African American and white adults: the Atherosclerosis Risk in Communities Study. JAMA 2000;283(17):2253–9.

54. American Diabetes Association Position Statement. Standards of medical care in diabetes - 2010. Diabetes Care 2010;33(Suppl 1):S11–61.

55. Borrell LN, Kunzel C, Lamster I, et al. Diabetes in the dental office: using NHANES III to estimate the probability of undiagnosed disease. J Periodont Res 2007;42(6): 559–65.

56. Strauss SM, Russell S, Wheeler A, et al. The dental office visit as a potential opportunity for diabetes screening: an analysis using NHANES 2003-2004 data. J Public Health Dent 2010;70(2):156–62.

57. Li S, Williams PL, Douglass CW. Development of a clinical guideline to predict undiagnosed diabetes in dental patients. J Am Dent Assoc 2011;142(1):28–37.

58. Lalla E, Kunzel C, Burkett S, et al. Identification of unrecognized diabetes and pre-diabetes in a dental setting. J Dent Res 2011;90(7):855–60.

59. Lin JW, Chang YC, Li HY, et al. Cross-sectional validation of diabetes risk scores for predicting diabetes, metabolic syndrome, and chronic kidney disease in Taiwanese. Diabetes Care 2009;32(12):2294–6.
60. Barasch A, Safford MM, Qvist V, et al. Random blood glucose testing in dental practice: a community-based feasibility study from the Dental Practice-Based Research Network. J Am Dent Assoc 2012;143(3):262–9.
61. Rosedale M, Strauss S. Diabetes screening at the periodontal visit: patient and provider experiences with two screening approaches. Int J Dent Hyg, 2011. Doi:10.1111/j.1601-5037.2011.00542.x [Epub ahead of print].
62. Hoerger TJ, Segel JE, Gregg EW, et al. Is glycemic control improving in U.S. adults? Diabetes Care 2008;31(1):81–6.

Obesity Prevention and Intervention in Dental Practice

Mary Tavares, DMD, MPH[a,b,*], Amanda Dewundara, BA[c],
J. Max Goodson, DDS, PhD[a]

KEYWORDS

- Obesity • Diabetes • Prevention • Oral health • Systemic health

KEY POINTS

- Dental professionals have an important role in the prevention and detection of many oral and systemic diseases because of their diagnostic and screening abilities, as well as the frequency of patient visits. These invaluable skills and practice paradigms should be considered as part of the equation to solve one of the largest public health concerns of our time: the obesity epidemic.
- There is a well-described connection between periodontal disease and diabetes, with implications that the relationship may be bi-directional. Periodontal disease and obesity are associated with inflammatory stress and increased production of proinflammatory cytokines. Clearly, these associations should be reasons for the dental profession to intervene in the rise of obesity.
- Insufficient sleep is another factor in the obesity problem and screening for sleep habits could be part of a comprehensive dental assessment, along with height, weight, blood pressure. The dental profession is in a unique position to identify and aid in the treatment of obstructive sleep apnea, a condition associated with obesity and diabetes.
- The rise of obesity and type 2 diabetes in children is of great concern and the dental profession can play a role in raising awareness of overweight status as well as obesity risk behaviors.

INTRODUCTION

Obesity is increasing at epidemic proportions in adults and in children on an international and national scale. The disturbing sequelae of this increased trajectory of overweight populations are the parallel increases in the chronic diseases that are comorbidities of obesity. According to the World Health Organization (WHO),

The authors have nothing to disclose.
[a] The Forsyth Institute, 245 First Street, Cambridge, MA 02142, USA; [b] Harvard School of Dental Medicine, 188 Longwood Avenue, Boston, MA 02115-5819, USA; [c] Columbia University College of Dental Medicine, 630 West 168th Street, New York, NY 10032, USA
* Corresponding author. The Forsyth Institute, 245 First Street, Cambridge, MA 02142.
E-mail address: mtavares@forsyth.org

Dent Clin N Am 56 (2012) 831–846
http://dx.doi.org/10.1016/j.cden.2012.07.009
0011-8532/12/$ – see front matter © 2012 Elsevier Inc. All rights reserved.

dental.theclinics.com

overweight and obesity can be defined as an abnormal or excessive level of fat accumulation that may impair health.[1] Like many chronic diseases, obesity has significant associated morbidity, mortality, and economic impact and is largely preventable.[2] Primary health care providers, including dental professionals, are well-positioned to address this public health problem at the patient level. It is increasingly evident that the dental profession is a stakeholder in the weight status of its patients and can be part of a coordinated effort to prevent and intervene in the obesity problem.

CAUSES AND FACTORS ASSOCIATED WITH OBESITY

Having multifactorial causes, obesity is largely attributed to the systemic energy imbalance created by excessive caloric intake and inadequate levels of physical activity. Since the 1970s, diets have shifted toward processed foods, greater use of edible oils, and the increased popularity of sugar-sweetened beverages. Furthermore, the advent of new technologies has allowed for a markedly more sedentary lifestyle.[3]

Some of the key factors associated with obesity risk include socioeconomic circumstances, minority status, geographic location, access to education, cultural beliefs, and genetic influences.[3] Generally, obesity and overweight conditions disproportionately affect Hispanic, African American, multiracial, and low-income populations.[4]

OBESITY INDICATORS IN ADULTS AND CHILDREN

Body mass index (BMI) is a useful, but imperfect measure to classify a population into categories based on height and weight status. In adults, a BMI of greater than or equal to 25 is considered overweight, and that greater than or equal to 30 is obese. These values are scaled the same for all ages and both genders.[5]

BMI percentiles are used to classify children. Values differ based on age and gender because the amount of body fat differs between males and females and changes with age. Overweight falls between the 85th and 94th percentile; obese are those greater than or equal to the 95th percentile.[5]

CURRENT STATISTICS
International

In 2010, WHO reported that approximately 43 million children younger than 5 were overweight, and that the distribution was no longer heavily skewed toward high-income countries. Nearly 35 million overweight children are living in parts of the developing world, and 8 million are in developed nations.[1] The same report states that 65% of the world's population lives in countries where overweight and obesity kill more people than underweight conditions. The onset of type 2 diabetes (T2DM) in young children has been falling in age and the prevalence of children ages 6 to 11 with T2DM had doubled in the past 20 years (**Fig. 1**).[6]

Internationally, it was estimated in 2008 that 1.5 billion adults, 20 and older, were overweight. Of these, over 200 million men and nearly 300 million women were obese. It was concluded that more than 1 in 10 of the global adult population is considered obese—a trend that has developed in the past decade.[1] **Fig. 2** display adult obesity (BMI >30) prevalence for selected countries around the world.[7,8] Rates are rising rapidly, particularly in African regions, Arab countries, and the United States.[1]

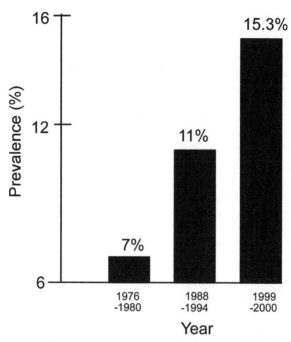

Fig. 1. The prevalence of type 2 diabetes in children in the United States. (*Data from* Gerberding JL. Diabetes, disabling disease to double by 2050. Centers for Disease Control and Prevention. 2007. Available at: http://www.cdc.gov/nccdphp/publications/aag/ddt.htm. Accessed April 8, 2012.)

National Epidemic and Trends

Children

As of 2010, 18% of children ages 6 to 11 and 18.4% of adolescents 12 to 19 were considered obese in the United States. This correlates with an overall 54.5% increase in children, and a 63.6% increase in adolescents since 2000.[9,10] Within the adolescent

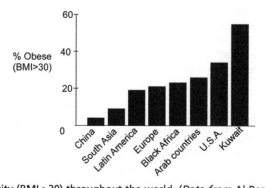

Fig. 2. Adult obesity (BMI >30) throughout the world. (*Data from* Al Rashdan I, Al Nesef Y. Prevalence of overweight, obesity, and metabolic syndrome among adult Kuwaitis: results from community-based national survey. Angiology 2010;61(1):42–8; and Flegal KM, Carroll MD, Ogden CL, et al. Prevalence and trends in obesity among US adults, 1999–2008. JAMA 2010;303(3):235–41.)

demographic, 13.9% meet the adult classification of obesity, with a BMI of 30 or greater.[10]

The childhood obesity trend has been rapidly increasing since 1980 and prevalence has nearly tripled in 20 years.[11] It is estimated that 30% of the young population in the United States will be obese by 2030.[12] Furthermore, a study by Ritchie and colleagues[13] found that a child who was overweight at any one point during the elementary school years was 25 times more likely to be overweight at age 12 than a child who was never previously overweight. It is predicted that 70% of overweight children will become obese adults with all the chronic disease implications attached,[14] which underscores the importance of early intervention efforts.

Adults

National Health and Nutrition Examination Survey (NHANES) results from 2009 to 2010 found that more than one-third of adults were obese, and there were no significant differences found between genders. In addition, adults 60 years or older were more likely to be obese than younger adults.[15] If the current trends continue, it is predicted that about 3 of 4 Americans will be overweight or obese by 2020.[16]

IMPACT
Burden of Disease

Obesity has both physical and psychological complications. Physiologically, it increases the risk of T2DM, sleep apnea, orthopedic complications, certain cancers,[16] periodontal disease (PD),[17] high blood lipids, hypertension, and other cardiovascular risk factors.[18,19] A recent study indicates that obesity may affect children before birth, linking maternal obesity and diabetes with autism spectrum disorder and developmental delays.[20] Psychosocially, obesity may have a long-term negative impact, leaving the patient vulnerable to the development of depression, anxiety, social isolation, discrimination, a lower quality of life, and stigmatization.[21] It has also been associated with unemployment, absenteeism, and the potential for lower wages in comparison with nonobese employees.[22]

Medical Costs

According to the Centers for Disease Control and Prevention, roughly $147 billion was devoted to obesity-related conditions in 2008. On average, the cost of health care for an obese individual exceeds that for a normal-weight person by $1429 per year.[23]

Total medical costs related to this condition are projected to double every decade to account for 16% to 18% of total US health care expenditure by 2030.[12] At this alarming rate, it is crucial for all health care providers to spread the message about the serious risks of obesity, and how it can be prevented with proper diet and lifestyle modifications.

THE RELATIONSHIP BETWEEN OBESITY AND ORAL HEALTH

Depending on how one reads the literature today, one may think of the obese dental patient as an individual with an extra set of risk factors that should be appreciated during their dental care. Or, one may think of PD as a condition that substantially contributes to obesity and should be controlled rigorously in patients who are obese or are at risk for developing obesity.

The association between obesity and cardiovascular disease[24] is well established. The association between PD and cardiovascular disease has also been extensively reviewed.[25] Although the literature in these fields is beyond the scope of obesity management in the dental office, they form an important background for its consideration.

PERIODONTAL DISEASE

It has long been recognized that PD is more prevalent in patients with T2DM[26–28] in whom obesity is a central attribute. In adults, PD is 3.1 times more likely to occur in overweight and 5.3 times more likely to occur in obese adults than in normal healthy weight adults and higher levels of the periodontal pathogen *Tannerella forsythia* was found more frequently in obese patients.[29]

At a simplistic level, the adipocytes of fat tissue, which are surprisingly active in metabolic regulation, produce both anti-inflammatory and proinflammatory mediators (**Fig. 3**). The inflammatory mediators released from PDs add to the adipocyte inflammatory mediators to enhance the systemic inflammatory state.

Periodontal therapy can reduce systemic inflammatory markers. For example, C-reactive protein (CRP) is reduced by periodontal treatment, which also has been shown to reduce serum levels of the proinflammatory cytokines leptin and interleukin-6.[30] However, this effect is nullified by the production of these same cytokines by the large number of adipocytes in obese individuals.[31]

Both diabetes and obesity are accentuated by PD. Thus, for example, blood levels of adiponectin, a hormone regulating glucose levels and fatty acid catabolism, are lower in patients with PD who also present with T2DM.[32,33] Gingival crevicular fluid levels of the proinflammatory cytokine tumor necrosis factor-α increase with BMI,[34] and metabolic syndrome has been shown to be more prevalent in patients with radiographic evidence of periodontal bone loss.[35,36] Obesity also increases the risk of having PD.[37] The generally proposed mechanism of this bilateral association is through their common ability to create oxidative (proinflammatory) stress.[38]

Upon acknowledging the common risk factors of obesity and PD, the question as to whether obesity causes PD or the converse has not been adequately answered.[28] Almost all studies conducted are cross-sectional, for which one cannot determine the directionality of association. The possibility that PD contributes to obesity is

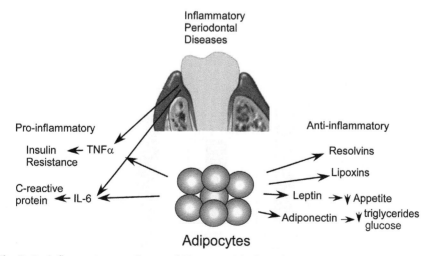

Fig. 3. Proinflammatory mediators of PDs sum with those from adipocytes to shift equilibrium to a predominately inflammatory state.

suggested by a prospective study that indicates that obesity develops more frequently in patients with periodontal pockets.[39] In this study, 1023 adults were selected who were not obese; 205 had periodontal pockets. Four years later, 22 (10.7%) of those who had pockets were obese as compared with 6.2% who did not have pockets. An odds ratio of 1.7 indicates that it is almost twice as likely to develop obesity if patients have PD at the outset. This difference approached statistical significance (P = .056). A similar comparison with missing teeth and dental caries was clearly not significant. These data are summarized in **Fig. 4.**

Both PD and obesity are associated with inflammatory stress and increased production of proinflammatory cytokines. Although an association seems to have been well established, there is no basis to recommend differences in dental treatment planning for obese patients[28] but there is reason to think that the dentist should be ready to participate in a weight management program for the overweight dental patient who may be adversely affected by their oral disease condition.

CHILDREN

Although it seems that children with gingivitis may be affected in the same manner as adults with periodontitis, far less periodontal research has been conducted with children.[40] In children, gingivitis occurs more frequently in obese children and is associated with insulin resistance.[41] Salivary flow rate is decreased and dental caries is increased in obese children.[42] Based on these observations, it appears that gingival inflammation may be the primary association between oral disease and obesity.

As previously noted, the incidence of child obesity has been escalating, and along with this trend is an increase in the prevalence of T2DM, as well as a lower age of onset. The same health behaviors affect adults and children: sedentary lifestyles and diets with excesses of fats and refined carbohydrates. These behaviors contribute to both obesity and T2DM. However, a link with obesity and dental caries has not been consistently found in studies (see section on caries and obesity).

INFECTOBESITY

It is possible that oral bacteria could have an effect on development of obesity. An animal model for bacterial induction of obesity has been described.[43–46] In this model, mice raised to be free of bacteria consume more food but gain less weight than

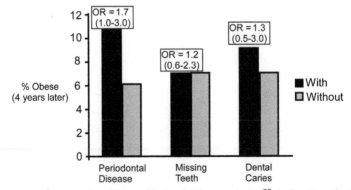

Fig. 4. A prospective study of the effect of PD on obesity[39] indicating that PD may contribute to the development of obesity. OR, odds ratio.

their wild-type brothers and sisters who become fat. Differences in gastrointestinal bacterial composition have been described. Similarly, reports have appeared that indicate oral bacteria in obese individuals differ from those of healthy normal weight.[47,48] It is appropriate to note that we all swallow about a gram (10^{11}) bacteria daily.[48]

SLEEP AND OBESITY

Sleep duration has been increasingly recognized as factor related to weight gain in children as well as adults.[49] In a study of 44,452 adults, those with sleep duration less than 6 hours were significantly more likely to meet metabolic syndrome criteria than those with longer sleep duration.[50] Sleep duration has been related to elevated blood pressure by several investigators.[51–55] There is sufficient evidence of association to the suggestion that sleep duration should be an important marker of cardiovascular disease.[54] In an experiment in which healthy young men were sleep restricted for just 2 days, Spiegel and colleagues[56] found decreased levels of the hormone leptin, which controls appetite, and a rise in plasma ghrelin levels, which increases appetite and favors the accumulation of lipids in visceral fatty tissue. In a more recent study of healthy individuals, Buxton and colleagues[57] reported that short and disrupted sleep altered insulin levels and slowed metabolism to a rate that could add more than 12 pounds of weight in a year.

Obstructive sleep apnea (OSA) is associated with both obesity and diabetes, and a summary review of multiple studies suggests that weight loss can improve OSA with a positive effect on metabolic and cardiovascular risks.[58] Among patients attending a diabetes obesity clinic, 58% had obstructive sleep apnea that was associated with worsening glycemic control.[59] Children are also affected by OSA. Kohler and colleagues[60] found that among adolescents, there was a 3.5-fold increase in OSA risk with each standard-deviation increase in BMI percentile. Studies have demonstrated a relationship between OSA, inflammation, and insulin resistance in obese as well as nonobese children.[61,62]

Dentists can play an active role in identifying children and adults with possible OSA and referring them for assessment.[63] Early detection, referral, and coordinated care with patients' physicians can prevent additional consequences and improve quality of life.[64] The increasing availability of oral appliances has resulted in more dentists becoming involved in the care of patients with sleep-related breathing disorders[65]; however, it is not clear if they are addressing weight status where appropriate.

CARIES AND OBESITY

Studies of the relationship between dental caries and BMI in children have not been conclusive. Most studies have not found a significant association between BMI for age and caries prevalence in primary or permanent dentition.[66,67] However, Hilgers and colleagues,[68] while confirming the lack of overall association, found that smooth surface caries increased significantly with BMI . There is evidence that overweight and obese children have accelerated dental development, which has implications for caries risk and orthodontic treatment.[69,70]

Dental caries and sleep duration were significantly related in a pilot study of ninety 10-year-old Kuwaiti girls. Those who reported shorter weekday sleep duration had more decayed and filled teeth surfaces and also reported consuming more sugars in a dietary survey.[71] Although multiple factors may contribute to this finding, one can speculate that the elevated levels of ghrelin that are associated with short sleep may contribute to sugar consumption.

A ROLE FOR THE DENTAL PROFESSION

It has been demonstrated that specific repeated messages from multiple sources are more likely to promote behavioral change than single-source messages.[72] Primary care physicians and pediatricians are well-equipped to address the obesity issue. The American Academy of Pediatrics recommends that health care providers should encourage healthy eating patterns and routine physical activity, and discourage TV and video time by providing families with education and anticipatory guidance.[73] However, evidence suggests that busy providers do not adequately follow these recommendations.[74] Several studies have found that the detection of obesity during routine medical appointments is low, and time constraints limit how much a clinician is willing or able to discuss with patients.[74–76] Perrin and colleagues[77] suggest that office-based tools targeting specific behaviors may be helpful. Dental professionals are in a good position to be able supplement and reinforce the information received in the medical setting, as well as to initiate the conversation. Tavares and Chomitz[78] developed and tested the feasibility of a dental office–based tool for children, targeting obesity risk behaviors. The *Healthy Weight Intervention*, based on the concepts of Motivational Interviewing[79,80] was designed for children of all weights and requires approximately 10 minutes during the routine hygiene visit. Using standard, evidence-based recommendations for improving obesity risks, this preventive intervention does not require specialized training.

The dental team is in a unique and favorable position to offer healthy weight intervention and obesity prevention. Most healthy patients visit a dentist more frequently than a physician on a yearly basis. Children and adolescents, in particular, follow the paradigm of annual medical and semiannual dental visits,[81] potentially allowing for twice the annual frequency of any intervention. Additionally, it is already standard practice for dental professionals to promote dietary habits that avoid calorie and sugar-dense foods and beverages as caries prevention. They can easily expand their counseling to emphasize the implications of these dietary practices, in addition to the positive effects of physical activity and other lifestyle changes, on both oral and systemic health. For patients with suspected weight issues, the dentist can work alongside pediatricians, family physicians, and dietitians by providing referrals.[81] Some dental settings, particularly pediatric dental practices, already measure weight and height for other purposes such as calculating dosages for local and general anesthesia.[81] Obtaining BMI and BMI percentile measurements can be a feasible addition to the dental protocol, as it is noninvasive, and requires a small time commitment and minimal cost.[82]

Accepting the premise that weight status is associated with oral health, weight screening, obesity prevention, and intervention in dental offices can be advocated as part of comprehensive dental assessment and treatment.[82] As previously discussed in this article, there are strong links between obesity and oral health, particularly with respect to diabetes and PD. Decreasing obesity risks through diet and lifestyle changes can have a positive impact on oral as well as systemic health. It is important for the dental team to consider all the key domains of obesity risk behaviors, such as physical activity, screen time, and meal patterns; not only diet (**Fig. 5**).[83]

Is the Dental Profession Ready and Willing?

An important study by Curran and colleagues[84] found that more than 50% of American Dental Association member dentists reported that they were interested in offering obesity-related services, but fewer than 5% did so. Interestingly, more than 60% of the general and pediatric dentists noted increases in overweight patients and 43%

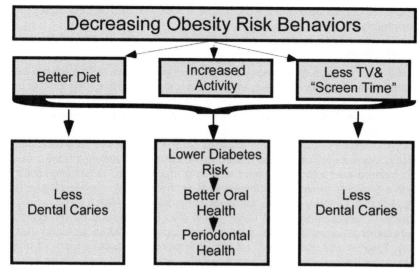

Fig. 5. Decreasing obesity risk factors can affect oral health.

of the general dentists reported diagnosing more gingival and periodontal problems in those patients. Eighty percent agreed that they would be more willing to address obesity if there was a definitive link with oral health. Curran and colleagues[84] report that the fear of offending patients or appearing too judgmental was the most reported barrier to considering obesity interventions. Additional barriers were lack of training and knowledge, time constraints, lack of reimbursement, and lack of coordinated services for referral.

A survey of North Carolina hygienists found that 95% felt that they have a role in helping patients improve nutrition and 65% were confident in discussing obesity-related risks.[85] Focus groups with dental hygienists have confirmed their willingness and confidence to expand their roles to include obesity prevention and intervention.[83]

Pediatric dentists have led the way in advocating and supporting the role of the dental profession in obesity management.[86] In the national survey of dentists, they were significantly more likely than general dentists to take a role in their patients' weight-related health care even without a connection with oral health.[84] Pediatric dentists report receiving nutritional and healthy lifestyle information during residency and continuing education programs, which may influence their confidence in broadening their scope of practice with their patients.[87]

Dental organizations have supported the role of the dental team in participating in obesity prevention. The American Academy of Pediatric Dentistry has set the monitoring, prevention, and management of childhood overweight as an important research agenda.[88] In 2005, the editor of the *Journal of the American Dental Association* expressed the view that dentists should institute and monitor obesity interventions; not only for the purposes of oral health, but for a desire to positively affect patients' general health.[89]

The concern that patients and their parents may be offended or opposed to dental-setting based interventions is not supported in the literature. Greenberg et al[90] reported that most inner-city patients in one study were willing to have a dentist screen them for systemic conditions and their opinions of dentists improved as a result. Parents of children in 2 studies of the *Healthy Weight Intervention* reported that their children were comfortable with the procedure and they agreed that the dental setting was appropriate.[91,92]

Future Directions

It is clear from surveys of dentists that education and exposure to systemic health interventions during training are key elements in encouraging the integration of these elements into clinical practice.[84,87] Therefore, introducing systemic health screenings, and prevention and intervention protocols to dental students is a key element in widespread implementation. Finding methods to work within the constraints of current practice modalities is important for feasibility. At the University of Toronto Faculty of Dentistry, students are using a simplified identification of overweight status in children[93] incorporated into a shortened version of the *Healthy Weight Intervention* to provide a 5-minute preventive intervention at each visit (S.M. Hashim Nainar, BDS, MDSc, Toronto, Ontario, Canada, personal communication, March 2012).

Expanding beyond the dental clinic, it will also be important to include dental delivery settings in schools that service lower-income children at higher risk for obesity. Tavares and colleagues[94] recently completed a feasibility study of obesity intervention in several models of school-based dental care. The conclusion was that integration of such an intervention requires additional time and the will to implement it. Parents and guardians welcomed the intervention and using the feedback sent home from their child's visit, reported making beneficial changes to their families' diets and meal patterns.[92]

Of all the obesity-related systemic diseases, diabetes has the most impact on the management of oral health. Identifying early cases or undiagnosed cases of T2DM in the dental setting would be a great service to patients and potentially affect the rising incidence and costs of this disease. Lalla and colleagues[95] proposed a predictive model using dental parameters for detection of undiagnosed diabetic individuals. Some dental sites, particularly in the absence of consistent medical care, conduct fingerstick blood glucose tests for their patients who are diabetic, irrespective of direct reimbursement (Krista Postai, Community Health Center of Southeast Kansas, Pittsburg, KS, personal communication, April 2012). Although blood tests are feasible in the dental setting, ultimately, the use of saliva as an early diagnostic tool for diabetes or its precursors would be a good fit for the dental profession.[96,97]

SUMMARY

Dental professionals have an important role in the prevention and detection of many oral and systemic diseases because of their diagnostic and screening abilities, as well as the frequency of patient visits. These invaluable skills and practice paradigms should be considered as part of the equation to solve one of the largest public health concerns of our time: the obesity epidemic. Currently, the United States and many other nations are in the midst of this epidemic and its resulting implications. Chronic diseases, particularly diabetes and cardiovascular disease, are the result of overweight conditions. There is a well-described connection between PD and diabetes, with implications that the relationship may be bi-directional. PD and obesity are associated with inflammatory stress and increased production of proinflammatory cytokines. Clearly, these associations should be reasons for the dental profession to intervene in the rise of obesity.

Insufficient sleep is another factor in the obesity problem and screening for sleep habits could be part of a comprehensive dental assessment, along with height, weight and blood pressure. The dental profession is in a unique position to identify and aid in the treatment of obstructive sleep apnea, a condition associated with obesity and diabetes.

The rise of obesity and T2DM in children is of great concern. Once again, the dental profession can play a role in raising awareness of overweight status as well as obesity risk behaviors.

Ultimately, a health condition as prevalent and serious as obesity must be approached by a concerted and collaborative effort of many disciplines and organizations. The dental profession should include itself in this collaboration, using the tools and education opportunities available. Although the connection between oral health and obesity is critical to understand, it should not be the sole motivating factor for taking action. As Glick stated in his appeal to raise the awareness of the dental profession with respect to obesity[89]: *"Direct participation in changing this health problem will not be simple, but is this not a challenge we should consider?"*

REFERENCES

1. World Health Organization. Obesity and overweight. Fact sheet No. 311, March 2011. Available at: http://www.who.int/mediacentre/factsheets/fs311/en/. Accessed April 7, 2012.
2. US Department of Health and Human Services. Centers for Disease Control and Prevention. The power of prevention: chronic disease—the public health challenge of the 21st century. 2009. Available at: http://www.cdc.gov/chronicdisease/pdf/2009-Power-of-Prevention.pdf. Accessed April 11, 2012.
3. Popkin BM, Adair LS, Ng SW. Global nutrition transition and the pandemic of obesity in developing countries. Nutr Rev 2012;70(1):3–21.
4. Skelton JA, Cook SR, Auinger P, et al. Prevalence and trends of severe obesity among US children and adolescents. Acad Pediatr 2009;9(5):322–9.
5. US Department of Health and Human Services. Centers for Disease Control and Prevention. Defining overweight and obesity. 2010. Available at: http://www.cdc.gov/obesity/defining.html. Accessed April 8, 2012.
6. Gerberding JL. Diabetes, disabling disease to double by 2050. Centers for Disease Control and Prevention; 2007. Available at: http://www.cdc.gov/nccdphp/publications/aag/ddt.htm. Accessed April 8, 2012.
7. Al Rashdan I, Al Nesef Y. Prevalence of overweight, obesity, and metabolic syndrome among adult Kuwaitis: results from community-based national survey. Angiology 2010;61(1):42–8.
8. Flegal KM, Carroll MD, Ogden CL, et al. Prevalence and trends in obesity among US adults, 1999-2008. JAMA 2010;303(3):235–41.
9. US Department of Health and Human Services. HHS releases assessment of Healthy People 2010 objectives. Life Expectancy Rises, but Health Disparities Remain. HHS News; 2011. Available at: www.healthypeople.gov/2020/about/HP2010PressReleaseOct5.doc. Accessed April 8, 2012.
10. Ogden CL, Carroll MD, Curtin LR, et al. Prevalence of high body mass index in US children and adolescents, 2007-2008. JAMA 2010;303(3):242–9.
11. US Department of Health and Human Services. Centers for Disease Control and Prevention. Overweight and obesity, data and statistics. April 2011. Available at: http://www.cdc.gov/obesity/childhood/data.html. Accessed April 8, 2012.
12. Wang Y, Beydoun MA, Liang L, et al. Will all Americans become overweight or obese? Estimating the progression and cost of the US obesity epidemic. Obesity (Silver Spring) 2008;16(10):2323–30.

13. Ritchie LD, Welk G, Styne D, et al. Family environment and pediatric overweight: what is a parent to do? J Am Diet Assoc 2005;105(5 Suppl 1):S70–9.

14. Serdula MK, Ivery D, Coates RJ, et al. Do obese children become obese adults? A review of the literature. Prev Med 1993;22(2):167–77.

15. Ogden CL, Carroll MD, Kit BK, et al. Prevalence of obesity in the united states, 2009-2010. NCHS Data Brief, No. 82. Hyattsville (MD): National Center for Health Statistics. Available at: http://www.cdc.gov/nchs/data/databriefs/db82.pdf. Accessed April 8, 2012.

16. Wang YC, McPherson K, Marsh T, et al. Health and economic burden of the projected obesity trends in the USA and the UK. Lancet 2011;378(9793):815–25.

17. Pischon N, Heng N, Bernimoulin JP, et al. Obesity, inflammation, and periodontal disease. J Dent Res 2007;86(5):400–9.

18. Schiel R, Beltschikow W, Kramer G, et al. Overweight, obesity and elevated blood pressure in children and adolescents. Eur J Med Res 2006;11(3):97–101.

19. Freedman DS, Dietz WH, Srinivasan SR, et al. The relation of overweight to cardiovascular risk factors among children and adolescents: the Bogalusa Heart Study. Pediatrics 1999;103(6 Pt 1):1175–82.

20. Krakowiak P, Walker CK, Bremer AA, et al. Maternal metabolic conditions and risk for autism and other neurodevelopmental disorders. Pediatrics 2012;129(5): e1121–8.

21. De Niet JE, Naiman DI. Psychosocial aspects of childhood obesity. Minerva Pediatr 2011;63(6):491–505.

22. Caliendo M, Lee WS. Fat chance! Obesity and the transition from unemployment to employment. Econ Hum Biol 2012. [Epub ahead of print].

23. US Department of Health and Human Services. Centers for Disease Control and Prevention. Overweight and obesity, economic consequences. 2011. Available at: http://www.cdc.gov/obesity/causes/economics.html. Accessed April 11, 2012.

24. Gray LJ, Cooper N, Dunkley A, et al. A systematic review and mixed treatment comparison of pharmacological interventions for the treatment of obesity. Obes Rev 2012;13(6):483–98.

25. Zelkha SA, Freilich RW, Amar S. Periodontal innate immune mechanisms relevant to atherosclerosis and obesity. Periodontol 2000 2010;54(1):207–21.

26. Rees TD. Periodontal management of the patient with diabetes mellitus. Periodontol 2000 2000;23:63–72.

27. Page RC, Offenbacher S, Schroeder HE, et al. Advances in the pathogenesis of periodontitis: summary of developments, clinical implications and future directions. Periodontol 2000 1997;14:216–48.

28. Chaffee BW, Weston SJ. Association between chronic periodontal disease and obesity: a systematic review and meta-analysis. J Periodontol 2010;81(12):1708–24.

29. Haffajee AD, Socransky SS. Relation of body mass index, periodontitis and *Tannerella forsythia*. J Clin Periodontol 2009;36(2):89–99.

30. Shimada Y, Komatsu Y, Ikezawa-Suzuki I, et al. The effect of periodontal treatment on serum leptin, interleukin-6, and C-reactive protein. J Periodontol 2010;81(8): 1118–23.

31. Offenbacher S, Beck JD, Moss K, et al. Results from the periodontitis and vascular events (PAVE) study: a pilot multicentered, randomized, controlled trial to study effects of periodontal therapy in a secondary prevention model of cardiovascular disease. J Periodontol 2009;80(2):190–201.

32. Hotta K, Funahashi T, Arita Y, et al. Plasma concentrations of a novel, adipose-specific protein, adiponectin, in type 2 diabetic patients. Arterioscler Thromb Vasc Biol 2000;20(6):1595–9.

33. Halleux CM, Takahashi M, Delporte ML, et al. Secretion of adiponectin and regulation of apM1 gene expression in human visceral adipose tissue. Biochem Biophys Res Commun 2001;288(5):1102–7.
34. Lundin M, Yucel-Lindberg T, Dahllof G, et al. Correlation between TNFalpha in gingival crevicular fluid and body mass index in obese subjects. Acta Odontol Scand 2004;62(5):273–7.
35. Nesbitt MJ, Reynolds MA, Shiau H, et al. Association of periodontitis and metabolic syndrome in the Baltimore Longitudinal Study of Aging. Aging Clin Exp Res 2010;22(3):238–42.
36. Alabdulkarim M, Bissada N, Al-Zahrani M, et al. Alveolar bone loss in obese subjects. J Int Acad Periodontol 2005;7(2):34–8.
37. Gorman A, Kaye EK, Apovian C, et al. Overweight and obesity predict time to periodontal disease progression in men. J Clin Periodontol 2012;39(2):107–14.
38. Bullon P, Morillo JM, Ramirez-Tortosa MC, et al. Metabolic syndrome and periodontitis: is oxidative stress a common link? J Dent Res 2009;88(6):503–18.
39. Morita T, Yamazaki Y, Mita A, et al. A cohort study on the association between periodontal disease and the development of metabolic syndrome. J Periodontol 2010; 81(4):512–9.
40. Bimstein E, Katz J. Obesity in children: a challenge that pediatric dentistry should not ignore—review of the literature. J Clin Pediatr Dent 2009;34(2):103–6.
41. Franchini R, Petri A, Migliario M, et al. Poor oral hygiene and gingivitis are associated with obesity and overweight status in paediatric subjects. J Clin Periodontol 2011;38(11):1021–8.
42. Modeer T, Blomberg CC, Wondimu B, et al. Association between obesity, flow rate of whole saliva, and dental caries in adolescents. Obesity (Silver Spring) 2010;18(12):2367–73.
43. Backhed F, Ding H, Wang T, et al. The gut microbiota as an environmental factor that regulates fat storage. Proc Natl Acad Sci U S A 2004;101(44):15718–23.
44. Backhed F, Ley RE, Sonnenburg JL, et al. Host-bacterial mutualism in the human intestine. Science 2005;307(5717):1915–20.
45. Backhed F, Manchester JK, Semenkovich CF, et al. Mechanisms underlying the resistance to diet-induced obesity in germ-free mice. Proc Natl Acad Sci U S A 2007;104(3):979–84.
46. Pasarica M, Dhurandhar NV. Infectobesity: obesity of infectious origin. Adv Food Nutr Res 2007;52:61–102.
47. Zeigler CC, Persson GR, Wondimu B, et al. Microbiota in the oral subgingival biofilm is associated with obesity in adolescence. Obesity (Silver Spring) 2012;20(1): 157–64.
48. Socransky SS, Haffajee AD. Dental biofilms: difficult therapeutic targets. Periodontol 2000 2002;28:12–55.
49. Patel SR, Hu FB. Short sleep duration and weight gain: a systematic review. Obesity (Silver Spring) 2008;16(3):643–53.
50. Kobayashi D, Takahashi O, Deshpande GA, et al. Association between weight gain, obesity, and sleep duration: a large-scale 3-year cohort study. Sleep Breath 2011. [Epub ahead of print].
51. Buxton OM, Marcelli E. Short and long sleep are positively associated with obesity, diabetes, hypertension, and cardiovascular disease among adults in the United States. Soc Sci Med 2010;71(5):1027–36.
52. Dean E, Bloom A, Cirillo M, et al. Association between habitual sleep duration and blood pressure and clinical implications: a systematic review. Blood Press 2012; 21(1):45–57.

53. Kim J, Jo I. Age-dependent association between sleep duration and hypertension in the adult Korean population. Am J Hypertens 2010;23(12):1286–91.
54. Sabanayagam C, Shankar A. Sleep duration and cardiovascular disease: results from the National Health Interview Survey. Sleep 2010;33(8):1037–42.
55. Wang H, Zee P, Reid K, et al. Gender-specific association of sleep duration with blood pressure in rural Chinese adults. Sleep Med 2011;12(7):693–9.
56. Spiegel K, Leproult R, L'Hermite-Baleriaux M, et al. Leptin levels are dependent on sleep duration: relationships with sympathovagal balance, carbohydrate regulation, cortisol, and thyrotropin. J Clin Endocrinol Metab 2004; 89(11):5762–71.
57. Buxton OM, Cain SW, O'Connor SP, et al. Adverse metabolic consequences in humans of prolonged sleep restriction combined with circadian disruption. Sci Transl Med 2012;4(129):129ra143.
58. Yu JC, Berger P 3rd. Sleep apnea and obesity. S D Med 2011;(Spec No):28–34.
59. Pillai A, Warren G, Gunathilake W, et al. Effects of sleep apnea severity on glycemic control in patients with type 2 diabetes prior to continuous positive airway pressure treatment. Diabetes Technol Ther 2011;13(9):945–9.
60. Kohler MJ, Thormaehlen S, Kennedy JD, et al. Differences in the association between obesity and obstructive sleep apnea among children and adolescents. J Clin Sleep Med 2009;5(6):506–11.
61. Verhulst SL, Schrauwen N, Haentjens D, et al. Sleep-disordered breathing and the metabolic syndrome in overweight and obese children and adolescents. J Pediatr 2007;150(6):608–12.
62. Verhulst SL, Schrauwen N, Haentjens D, et al. Sleep-disordered breathing in overweight and obese children and adolescents: prevalence, characteristics and the role of fat distribution. Arch Dis Child 2007;92(3):205–8.
63. Padmanabhan V, Kavitha PR, Hegde AM. Sleep disordered breathing in children—a review and the role of a pediatric dentist. J Clin Pediatr Dent 2010; 35(1):15–21.
64. Simmons MS, Clark GT. The potentially harmful medical consequences of untreated sleep-disordered breathing: the evidence supporting brain damage. J Am Dent Assoc 2009;140(5):536–42.
65. Mohsenin N, Mostofi MT, Mohsenin V. The role of oral appliances in treating obstructive sleep apnea. J Am Dent Assoc 2003;134(4):442–9.
66. Vann WF Jr, Bouwens TJ, Braithwaite AS, et al. The childhood obesity epidemic: a role for pediatric dentists? Pediatr Dent 2005;27(4):271–6.
67. Macek MD, Mitola DJ. Exploring the association between overweight and dental caries among US children. Pediatr Dent 2006;28(4):375–80.
68. Hilgers KK, Akridge M, Scheetz JP, et al. Childhood obesity and dental development. Pediatr Dent 2006;28(1):18–22.
69. Hilgers KK, Kinane DE, Scheetz JP. Association between childhood obesity and smooth-surface caries in posterior teeth: a preliminary study. Pediatr Dent 2006; 28(1):23–8.
70. Must A, Phillips SM, Tybor DJ, et al. The association between childhood obesity and tooth eruption. Obesity (Silver Spring) 2012. [Epub ahead of print].
71. Tavares M, Goodson JM, Cugini M, et al. Kuwait healthy lifestyle study: sleep as a health factor. Abstract #514. Tampa (FL): AADR; 2012.
72. Friedman SR, Des Jarlais DC, Sotheran JL. AIDS health education for intravenous drug users. Health Educ Q 1986;13(4):383–93.
73. American Academy of Pediatrics Committee on Nutrition. Prevention of pediatric overweight and obesity. Pediatrics 2003;112(2):424–30.

74. O'Brien SH, Holubkov R, Reis EC. Identification, evaluation, and management of obesity in an academic primary care center. Pediatrics 2004;114(2):e154–9.
75. Barlow SE, Dietz WH, Klish WJ, et al. Medical evaluation of overweight children and adolescents: reports from pediatricians, pediatric nurse practitioners, and registered dietitians. Pediatrics 2002;110(1 Pt 2):222–8.
76. Larsen L, Mandleco B, Williams M, et al. Childhood obesity: prevention practices of nurse practitioners. J Am Acad Nurse Pract 2006;18(2):70–9.
77. Perrin EM, Finkle JP, Benjamin JT. Obesity prevention and the primary care pediatrician's office. Curr Opin Pediatr 2007;19(3):354–61.
78. Tavares M, Chomitz V. A healthy weight intervention for children in a dental setting: a pilot study. J Am Dent Assoc 2009;140(3):313–6.
79. Resnicow K, Davis R, Rollnick S. Motivational interviewing for pediatric obesity: conceptual issues and evidence review. J Am Diet Assoc 2006;106(12):2024–33.
80. Schwartz RP, Hamre R, Dietz WH, et al. Office-based motivational interviewing to prevent childhood obesity: a feasibility study. Arch Pediatr Adolesc Med 2007; 161(5):495–501.
81. Tseng R, Vann WF Jr, Perrin EM. Addressing childhood overweight and obesity in the dental office: rationale and practical guidelines. Pediatr Dent 2010;32(5): 417–23.
82. Hague AL, Touger-Decker R. Weighing in on weight screening in the dental office: practical approaches. J Am Dent Assoc 2008;139(7):934–8.
83. Tavares M, Chomitz V, Cabral H, et al. Healthy weight intervention for children: feasibility in a dental setting. Abstract #0009. New Orleans (LA): IADR; 2007.
84. Curran AE, Caplan DJ, Lee JY, et al. Dentists' attitudes about their role in addressing obesity in patients: a national survey. J Am Dent Assoc 2010;141(11): 1307–16.
85. Kading CL, Wilder RS, Vann WF Jr, et al. Factors affecting North Carolina dental hygienists' confidence in providing obesity education and counseling. J Dent Hyg 2010;84(2):94–102.
86. Grossi SG, Collier DN, Perkin RM. Association of Medical School Pediatric Department Chairs I. Integrating oral health to the care of overweight children: a model of care whose time has come. J Pediatr 2008;152(4):451–2, 452.e1.
87. Braithwaite AS, Vann WF Jr, Switzer BR, et al. Nutritional counseling practices: how do North Carolina pediatric dentists weigh in? Pediatr Dent 2008;30(6): 488–95.
88. AAPD. American Academy of Pediatric Dentistry Research Agenda, 2007. Available at: http://www.aapd.org/media/policies_guidelines/researchagenda.pdf. Accessed April 10, 2012.
89. Glick M. A concern that cannot weight. J Am Dent Assoc 2005;136(5):572–4.
90. Greenberg BL, Kantor ML, Jiang SS, et al. Patients' attitudes toward screening for medical conditions in a dental setting. J Public Health Dent 2012;72(1): 28–35.
91. Tavares M, Chomitz V, Cabral H, et al. Acceptability and feasibility of obesity prevention in a dental office. Abstract # 0011. Dallas (TX): AADR; 2008.
92. Dewundara A, Tavares M, Chomitz V, et al. Attitudes regarding healthy weight counseling in a school-based dental setting. Abstract # 2589. San Diego (CA): IADR; 2011.
93. Nainar SM. Identification of overweight in children in the United States: a simplified approach. Obesity (Silver Spring) 2012;20(4):819–29.
94. Tavares M, Dewundara A, Chomitz V, et al. Feasibility of obesity prevention in school-based dental programs. Abstract # 471. San Diego (CA): IADR; 2011.

95. Lalla E, Kunzel C, Burkett S, et al. Identification of unrecognized diabetes and pre-diabetes in a dental setting. J Dent Res 2011;90(7):855–60.
96. Hasturk H, Goodson JM, Cugini M, et al. Kuwait healthy life study: salivary biomarkers in 10-year old children. Abstract #513. Tampa (FL): AADR; 2012.
97. Tremblay M, Gaudet D, Brisson D. Metabolic syndrome and oral markers of cardiometabolic risk. J Can Dent Assoc 2011;77:b125.

Identification of the Risk for Osteoporosis in Dental Patients

Hugh Devlin, PhD, MSc, BDS

KEYWORDS

- Osteoporosis • Risk factors • Implant survival • Periodontal disease

KEY POINTS

- Osteoporosis can be diagnosed using clinical questionnaires that attempt to identify those who have strong risk factors for the disease. Lifestyle factors such as the excessive use of alcohol and smoking are known to be risk factors for osteoporosis.
- Osteoporosis can be diagnosed through an analysis of the sparse trabeculation and thinning of the mandibular cortex often seen in dental panoramic radiographs.
- As a result of the radiographic and clinical findings, the dentist may suspect a patient has an increased risk of osteoporotic fractures and refer them for further tests, preventive advice, and treatment.
- There is no evidence that osteoporosis initiates periodontal disease. The role of osteoporosis in periodontal disease is unclear as there are many conflicting reports, but the evidence suggests that tooth loss may be more prevalent in patients with osteoporosis.
- There is no evidence that osteoporosis affects the clinical success rate of dental implants.

OSTEOPOROSIS ASSESSMENT TOOLS

Osteoporosis is a disease characterized by a severe loss of bone mineral density that can eventually result in fracture. The femur and spine are most commonly affected, and bone density measurements at these sites are expressed as T-score values. These values are the number of standard deviations by which the bone mineral density value lies below the sex-matched young adult value. Therefore as the T score becomes more negative, the patient is judged to be more severely affected by osteoporosis. According to the World Health Organization (WHO), patients with a T score of less than −2.5 are osteoporotic, whereas those with a T score between −1 and −2.5 have a bone mineral density less than normal and are osteopenic.[1]

The sensitivity of a test measures the proportion of people with osteoporosis that the test can correctly identify, whereas specificity provides a measure of a test's ability to correctly identify healthy people who do not have osteoporosis. By plotting sensitivity against (1 − specificity), the diagnostic accuracy of the test can be calculated as

School of Dentistry, University of Manchester, Higher Cambridge St, Manchester M15 6FH, UK
E-mail address: Hugh.Devlin@Manchester.ac.uk

Dent Clin N Am 56 (2012) 847–861
http://dx.doi.org/10.1016/j.cden.2012.07.010
0011-8532/12/$ – see front matter © 2012 Elsevier Inc. All rights reserved.

dental.theclinics.com

the area under the curve, a technique called receiver-operating characteristic curve (ROC) analysis. A test with a value of 0.5 has no diagnostic ability, and the accuracy of the test increases as the ROC value approaches unity.

RISK FACTORS

The presence of osteoporosis and the likelihood that an individual will develop a fracture can be identified.[2] Numerous assessment tools have been developed based on the patient's risk factors, namely body weight, age, current estrogen use, rheumatoid arthritis, ethnicity, and a history of nontraumatic fracture, and these tools have been compared against the WHO gold-standard diagnosis of osteoporosis. None of these tests are sufficiently accurate to provide a confirmatory diagnosis of osteoporosis. Rather, their purpose is to identify those people at increased risk of an osteoporotic hip fracture so that interceptive therapy can be given. However, opinion is divided as to where to place the diagnostic threshold. If the objective is to obtain a test with maximum sensitivity, this result in a large number of inappropriate false-positive referrals. The patients who are affected have to undergo needless worry. In addition, the referral of significant numbers of healthy individuals uses scant health care resources and is not cost effective. Conversely, using a high-specificity and low-sensitivity threshold will result in a failure to identify many women with osteoporosis, a proportion of whom will develop hip fractures in the future.

Dentists can use information from the patient's dental panoramic radiograph and an assessment of their clinical risk factors to determine whether they are at risk of osteoporosis. It is not recommended that a radiograph is taken specifically for an osteoporosis diagnosis, because the test is not as accurate as the medical criterion test, but it is quick and convenient for the patient.

In a large study population of 7779 women in the United States, Gourlay and colleagues[3] found that body weight had an area under the ROC curve of 0.73 (95% confidence interval [CI] 0.72–0.75) in identifying low bone density in women aged 67 years and older. The use of multiple clinical risk factors has been used to improve the osteoporosis diagnostic tool. Combinations of clinical factors such as age, weight, use of hormone replacement therapy, and a history of low trauma fracture are used in the Osteoporosis Index of Risk (OSIRIS) index.[4] Karayianni and colleagues[5] analyzed 653 women aged 45 to 70 years and showed that OSIRIS had an area under the ROC curve of 0.83 (95% CI 0.81–0.87) in detecting osteoporosis at either the hip, femoral neck, or spine.

Radiographic Changes in Dental Panoramic Radiographs

The inferior cortical border of the mandible is thinned in osteoporosis, and this can be detected on panoramic radiographs. Where a thin mandibular cortex is visible, the dentist should investigate the clinical risk factors to determine whether the patient should be referred for further investigation and diagnosis.

Fig. 1A illustrates the clearly distinct outline of the normal inferior mandibular cortex. **Fig. 1**B shows the indistinct endosteal border of the mandibular cortex in a patient with osteoporosis of the hip. Such a radiographic finding is often, but not always, observed. **Fig. 1**C is a more detailed image of this region showing the multiple layered appearance and porous nature of the cortex. A series of patchy radiopaque "residues" are

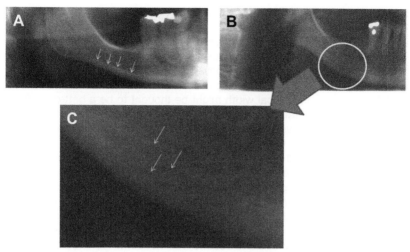

Fig. 1. (*A*) The clearly distinct outline of the normal inferior mandibular cortex (*arrows*). (*B*) The indistinct endosteal border of the mandibular cortex in a patient with osteoporosis of the hip. (*C*) A more detailed image of this region showing the multiple layered appearance (*arrows*) and porous nature of the cortex. Note also a series of patchy radiopaque "residues", representing the remains of the resorbed cortex that now form an intermediate, coarsely structured cancellous bone.

also seen, representing the remains of the resorbed cortex that now form an intermediate, coarsely structured cancellous bone.

Can dental radiographs be used to identify patients with osteoporosis?

Roberts and colleagues[6] evaluated the change in mandibular cortical width in 4949 dental panoramic tomograms of patients aged 15 to 94 years. In women, there was no change in cortical width during adulthood until age 42.5 years, when bone loss accelerated thereafter. This pattern of cortical thinning also occurs in the hip,[7] where it may result in weakening and bone fracture following trauma.

If dentists are to be more involved in proactively identifying those with osteoporosis, patients with mandibular cortical thinning should be referred to their physician for further investigation. Accurate measurement of the cortical width can be difficult, given the indistinct nature of the endosteal cortical border (see **Fig. 1**); therefore Horner and colleagues[8] proposed a 3-mm threshold as a compromise between detecting the maximum number of "true" osteoporotic patients and avoiding unnecessarily alarming patients who were subsequently found to have a normal bone density. This approach produced low sensitivity (8%) at detecting osteopenia at either the hip or spine, but specificity was high (98.7%). Others have proposed higher cortical-width thresholds. Lee and colleagues[9] used a threshold of 3.9 mm, and found a sensitivity of 72.9% and specificity of 70.2% in detecting low bone mineral density at the femoral neck. Using this higher threshold increased the sensitivity of the osteoporosis detection method, but decreased the specificity. Damilakis and Vlasiadis[10] found that a threshold of 4.1 mm produced sensitivity of 58.8% and specificity of 66.7% at detecting patients with osteoporosis at either the lumbar spine or the hip. Taguchi and colleagues[11] found that a cortical-width threshold of 4.3 mm produced sensitivity of 90% and specificity of 45.3% for identifying women with osteoporosis. Whatever the threshold chosen, the main conclusion from these studies is that a dental panoramic radiograph is not justified solely for the purposes of triage screening for osteoporosis, because of the high percentage of false positives that would result. But when a radiograph is taken for unrelated reasons and the dentist makes an incidental finding of cortical thinning and porosity, the patient may be at high risk of osteoporosis, and a referral to the patient's physician may be indicated.

The mandible is composed of 2 thick cortical plates with a sandwich of cancellous bone. At first glance, the cortical width might be thought to be a better predictor of osteoporosis at the femoral neck than at the lumbar spine, given the highly cortical nature of the former. However, there is no clear evidence for a difference in the detection rate of osteoporosis at the 2 sites.[12]

Other studies have found that a sparse cancellous bone pattern in the mandibular premolar region is associated with an increased number of self-reported fractures.[13] This pattern is seen as large intertrabecular spaces in the interdental area of the mandible. The loss of connectedness of the cancellous architecture in the mandible may reflect a similar general pattern of bone loss elsewhere in the aging skeleton.

Future research is also needed to identify those factors that may influence a patient's access to osteoporosis diagnosis and treatment services when referred by the dentist; for example, the support of the physician, the available resources, the type of health care system, the patient's consent, and the remuneration system offered to the dentist. Diagnosis of a patient's risk of osteoporosis will increasingly use computer-assisted diagnosis to automatically detect the cortices on the panoramic radiograph, measure cortical width, and alert the dentist as to whether the patient has a high risk of osteoporosis.[14] Such computer software already exists, and also allows data from the cortical-width measurements to be combined with clinical risk factors to produce a powerful diagnostic tool.[5]

Clinical Risk Factors for Osteoporosis

The major and minor risk factors for osteoporosis are listed in **Table 1**. One of the main risk factors is a low body weight or body mass index (BMI).

> A low body weight is a strong risk factor for osteoporosis. Those young women with anorexia nervosa are at an increased risk of premenopausal osteoporosis. Rapid bone loss occurs early, but bone density increases following weight gain.

Are those with osteoporosis more likely to suffer from periodontal disease?

Periodontal disease is triggered by plaque and poor dental hygiene. As periodontal bone loss can continue in some patients despite good oral-hygiene practices, many have considered whether osteoporosis could be a significant risk factor for periodontal disease. Osteoporosis causes a reduction in bone mass throughout the

Table 1
Clinical risk factors for osteoporosis

Major Clinical Risk Factors	Less Important Clinical Risk Factors
Old age	Dementia
Low body weight	High alcohol intake
Ovariectomy at an early age	Little physical activity
Previous low-impact bone fracture	
Rheumatoid arthritis and corticosteroids	

body, and the increased porosity of the alveolar bone surrounding the teeth may make it less resistant to resorption with plaque-induced inflammation. Unfortunately, most of the studies are cross-sectional in design and definitive conclusions are often not possible because of the small sample sizes. Pilgram and colleagues[15] examined 135 patients, and found weak correlations between clinical attachment loss and bone mineral density. A larger study involving 778 subjects, about half (53%) of whom were women, found a weak association between osteoporosis and periodontitis in women (crude odds ratio [OR] 1.8, 95% CI 1.1–3.3).[16]

Cross-sectional studies can be used to study risk factors (eg, osteoporosis) on an outcome (eg, periodontal disease or tooth loss), but this design is weak. To minimize bias, the assessment of the outcome must be blinded to prognostic information. Most studies comparing osteoporosis and periodontal disease are retrospective analyses of databases. When determining whether osteoporosis is an important prognostic factor in determining tooth loss, it is important to adjust for other prognostic variables, for example, oral hygiene and smoking. Multiple regression analysis is therefore usually required, but when comparing these studies investigators have included a variety of different variables. Could a declining alveolar bone density and osteoporosis account for the increased number of teeth lost by elderly women in some surveys? Tooth loss is the result of many social and clinical factors that interact in a complicated way, and it is difficult to isolate the effect of osteoporosis. The patient's caries and periodontal disease, as well as attitude and personal finance issues, are often the main factors in determining whether a patient has a tooth removed.

One of the first early studies found a low, but statistically significant, correlation between the periodontal index of posterior teeth and osteoporosis of the metacarpal bone,[17] although the smoking status of the patients was not assessed. Other studies have found a small additional effect of osteoporosis, even after adjustment for smoking and age. Both smoking and increasing age have a negative effect on both osteoporosis and periodontal disease. The methods of assessing the severity and extent of periodontal disease and osteoporosis in these studies vary widely, with consequently a large variation in the comparison groups.

There is general agreement in the literature that osteoporosis does not initiate periodontal disease, but there is considerable controversy as to whether osteoporosis can accelerate the progression of periodontal disease. Kribbs[18] examined 85 women with osteoporosis and 27 normal women, and found no difference in the periodontal measurements between the 2 groups. The women with osteoporosis had a history of vertebral compression fractures, but the severity of the osteoporosis or bone mass at this site was not available. If osteoporosis has a small effect on the progression of periodontal disease, the effect is more likely to be observed in the severely osteoporotic elderly. Von Wowern and colleagues[19] found that a group of osteoporotic women had a significantly lower bone mineral content in their forearm compared with a control group, and there was a significantly greater loss of periodontal attachment in the osteoporotic women, but no differences were found with respect to plaque score and gingival bleeding.

Osteoporosis does not initiate periodontal disease. Its role, if any, in aggravating preexisting periodontal disease is controversial.

In a study by Elders and colleagues,[20] no correlation was seen between the mean probing depth and the lumbar spine bone mineral density in a sample of 286 women, of whom 60 (21%) were edentulous. Only premenopausal or perimenopausal women were studied, as only those aged 46 to 55 years were included. Studies involving younger women are unlikely to involve severely affected osteoporotic individuals, as osteoporosis is mainly a disease of the elderly. Despite this, Taikaishi and colleagues[21] found an association between alveolar bone mineral density and periodontal pocket depth in a sample of 40 perimenopausal and postmenopausal women aged 50 to 69 years. Direct evidence for a causal relationship between declining estrogen levels and reduced alveolar bone density was found in the more porous alveolar bone of ovariectomized monkeys.[22] The less dense alveolar bone may be more prone to periodontal disease.[23]

Many of the population studies were not conducted in populations being seen specifically for dental services. For example, Gomes-Filho and colleagues[24] examined patients attending a reproduction assistance program. In the group with periodontal disease, 139 (83.3%) postmenopausal women had a very high prevalence of osteoporosis or osteopenia, compared with those with no periodontal disease (65.9%). Other studies are ancillary studies of large osteoporotic fracture studies, for example, the Pittsburgh Clinical Center for the Study of Osteoporotic Fractures.[25] In this 2-year longitudinal study, no difference in hip bone mineral density was found between women with and without periodontal disease. Differences in the assessment of periodontal disease, skeletal bone density, and age group studied limit any comparison between studies. Inagaki and colleagues[26] used a community-based Oral Health Screening Program to recruit 101 postmenopausal women. The investigators assessed the patients' osteoporotic status by means of computed densitometry of the metacarpal bone, and did not use the WHO classification. The age-adjusted odds of having fewer than 20 teeth were greater among those postmenopausal women with a very low bone mineral density in comparison with the normal group (OR = 5.9). However, the 95% CIs for this were wide (1.2–28.6), indicating that a larger sample size is required. Nineteen women were present in the very low bone mineral density group, of whom 6 had fewer than 20 teeth. The odds of tooth loss and periodontal disease were significantly higher in postmenopausal Japanese women with reduced metacarpal bone mineral density. Statistical adjustment for smoking status and prevalence of teeth with caries and restorations did not affect the relationship between severity of periodontal disease and metacarpal bone density.[26]

In a multicenter study funded by the European Union (Osteodent Study), 665 women aged 45 to 70 years were recruited. Bone density was measured at the total hip, femoral neck, and lumbar spine. On average, the osteoporotic subjects had about 3 fewer teeth than normal subjects. If those with edentulousness are excluded, the osteoporotic group had a mean of about 2 fewer teeth. After adjusting for age, smoking, and center, there was a significant association between osteoporosis and having fewer than 28 teeth remaining ($P = .011$), which may indicate that osteoporosis has an effect on particular tooth groups (eg, molar teeth rather than anterior teeth).[27]

Astrom and colleagues[28] examined the dental status of 14,375 individuals in a Swedish community. For both men and women the incidence of fracture was correlated with the degree of tooth loss, but the statistical relationship of both factors is not proof of a causative relationship. There is an increasing tooth loss and bone fracture incidence with age, but both may be occurring independently. However, in this study, in those older than 70 years women generally had a fewer mean number of teeth at each age than men. In most studies, it is a small minority of the study population that accounts for the majority of the tooth loss.

In a cross-sectional study, Bollen and colleagues[29] reported no significant difference in the number of teeth between those with and without bone fractures. Patients were asked to recall their previous fractures, and this potentially selective recall may have introduced error. May and colleagues[30] found a significant association in 608 men and 874 women, aged 65 to 76 years, between the bone mineral density at the hip and spine and the patients' self-reported tooth loss. Adjustment for confounding variables such as age and cigarette smoking did not alter the result. It is not known whether any misclassification of self-reported tooth number produced a random error in this study. The investigators argued that if all patients were inconsistent in stating how many teeth they had lost, a random error would result that would add variability to the data, and no significant association would have resulted. In this study, no information was provided on how these patients had lost their teeth. Trauma, caries, and periodontal disease are usually the main contributing factors to the number of teeth lost by patients. These factors are active throughout life, unlike a low bone mineral density, which usually develops only later in life. Klemetti and Vainio[31] reported no association between tooth loss and bone mineral density at the hip and lumbar spine. Similarly, Earnshaw and colleagues[32] found no relationship between tooth count and bone mineral density in early postmenopausal women.

Krall and colleagues[33] found that systemic bone loss predicted tooth loss in a sample of 189 postmenopausal women aged 41 to 71 years in a 7-year prospective study. Subjects in this study were included if they had a normal spinal bone mineral density and a low dietary calcium intake, but this may mean that the study participants were unrepresentative of the general population of women from the United States. The number of teeth lost during the study was assessed by questionnaire, which may have also introduced some measurement error. There were no measurements in the sample of periodontal disease status and no investigation of the reasons for the tooth loss.

Yoshihara and colleagues[34] examined 600 people aged 70 years, and found a significant relationship between the number of remaining teeth and bone mineral density of the os calcis. In this study, measurement at the os calcis was undertaken using ultrasound densitometry, which is not considered to be the gold-standard measurement technique for bone mineral density. This study demonstrated a clinically significant reduction of 2 to 3 teeth when comparing the mean tooth number for the female osteopenia group (15.97, SD = 9.98) with that of the control group (18.31, SD = 8.06). However, given the large standard deviation associated with the number of teeth, it would not be accurate to say to an individual patient with osteoporosis that they would be likely to lose a further 2 to 3 teeth as a result of this disease.

The United Kingdom Adult Dental Health Survey[35] has shown that women have fewer sound and untreated teeth than do men. Osteoporosis may be the cause of this difference, as women are more frequently affected by osteoporosis. Alternatively, women may be more demanding about aesthetics and request the extraction of irregular teeth. The latter explanation would predict that more elderly women than men of the same age have missing anterior teeth, but have a similar mean number of posterior teeth.

A prospective cohort study of 1341 recruited postmenopausal women were followed up for a mean of 5.1 years[36] to investigate the factors predisposing to tooth loss. Preexisting periodontal disease, plaque, a history of smoking, diabetes, and previous missing teeth at the baseline examination were all important in predicting future tooth loss. A lower BMI is associated with osteoporosis, but in this study a higher BMI was associated with an increased incidence of tooth loss. The effect was small (about one tooth on average was lost for a 5 kg/m^2 increase in BMI). In a longitudinal 5-year study involving postmenopausal Japanese women, Iwasaki and colleagues[37] found that those with the greater reduction in bone mineral density over this period were more likely to lose teeth, although the effect was small. The relative risk for the highest tertile percentage change from baseline bone density was 1.38 (95% CI

1.11–1.72) for the lumbar spine and 1.27 (95% CI 1.01–1.59) for the femoral neck. The result remained significant after controlling for menopausal age, high alcohol consumption, vitamin D and calcium intake, BMI, and diabetes. Smokers were excluded from the study.

In research there tends to be a bias against publishing studies that show no statistically significant effects, so it can be difficult to assess the true association between variables. Studies that do not show any association between variables or any benefit of a particular drug intervention tend to remain unpublished. There are, of course, exceptions to this general statement. For example, in a Japanese cross-sectional study, there was no significant difference in the number of teeth remaining between those who used estrogen and those who did not.[38] There are studies showing the opposite, that is, a positive beneficial effect of estrogen replacement on tooth loss.[39]

In conclusion, there is some evidence for a small clinical effect of osteoporosis on increasing tooth loss. However, further laboratory investigations are required to provide a biological mechanism of action that will, in turn, supply a clinically testable hypothesis.

Do oral implants have less success when used in osteoporotic patients?

Many factors interact to determine the success rate of oral implants. The failure rate of this form of treatment is very low; therefore if the effect of a factor on the rate of implant success is to be determined, the studies must be large and therefore expensive. However, if a very large study is required to demonstrate a small statistically significant effect, the clinical importance of that factor must also be separately considered. When considering the published studies, the question has to be asked whether other potentially more influential factors have been accounted for in the analysis or in the experimental methodology. Lee and colleagues[40] concluded, in a retrospective study, that implant treatment should not be considered to be a particularly high-risk procedure for older patients with controlled systemic conditions. However, they collected data from only 35 patients who were followed for a mean period of only 32.7 months. If a dental implant is placed in cancellous bone that has sparse trabeculation and is of low density, it will provide poor support for an implant in function and may result in its loss. Glauser and colleagues[41] found that only two-thirds of implants placed in the posterior maxilla were successful, probably because of the low-density bone that is usually found in this region.

The importance of the density of the host bone is well known in orthopedic surgery. In the older osteoporotic patient with a hip fracture, the bone quality is extremely important in determining the success or failure of internal fixation. Complications of hip-fracture fixation are common. Where bone support is critically low, the surgeon may be unable to place any internal fixation device. The Singh index[42] has been used in assessment of femoral trabecular bone structure, but has the disadvantage that there is considerable interobserver variability with its use.

CLINICAL STUDIES IN OSTEOPOROTIC PATIENTS RECEIVING IMPLANT TREATMENT

In a retrospective study[43] of 192 women aged at least 50 years at the time of implant placement, there was no increased risk of implant failure in those with osteoporosis and osteopenia. In the same study, those patients who smoked cigarettes at the time of implant placement suffered more implant failures; the implants were 2.6 times more likely to fail than those placed in nonsmokers.

Most clinical studies show that implant therapy is a successful treatment in patients with osteoporosis. Friberg and colleagues[44] placed implants in a small sample of 16 patients with osteoporosis or osteopenia of the spine or the hip, or both. Only

2 implants failed. A larger study[45] compared the success rate of endosseous implants in 168 postmenopausal women not receiving estrogen replacement therapy and in 75 postmenopausal women taking estrogen. Patients with other metabolic bone disease were excluded from the study, as were those who smoked or used alcohol. Patients in the unsupplemented postmenopausal group suffered more frequent maxillary implant failure compared with the younger premenopausal group. Of implants placed in this older group, 13.6% (78 of 302) failed compared with 6.3% (7 of 112) in the younger group. However, both groups underwent a high frequency of maxillary implant failure, with no bone-grafting methodology described.

Amorim and colleagues[46] found no difference in the success rate of implants placed in a control group and a group with osteoporosis of the lumbar spine and femoral neck. Indeed, there was a more frequent loss of bone from the alveolar bone crest in control subjects than in the osteoporotic group. Thirty-nine implants were placed in the 19 patients from the osteoporotic group, and 43 implants were placed in the 20 individuals from the control group. Of the 82 implants placed, only 1 failed. The failed implant occurred in the osteoporotic patient, but there was no evidence that osteoporosis impeded implant osseointegration.

In a retrospective study involving a group of women older than 50 years, Holahan and colleagues[43] found that patients with osteoporosis or osteopenia were not more likely to experience implant failure. Patients with osteoporosis had a 93% implant success rate of the 143 implants placed; those with osteopenia had a 94.9% success rate with 197 implants placed; and those in the control group a 94.4% success rate with 306 implants placed. Osteoporosis was not found to be associated with either a failure of implants to osseointegrate or a failure of existing osseointegration. In this study, the osteoporotic status of patients was obtained from measurements of the spine, femoral neck, and radius (although 90.6% of the measurements used the spine). As the bone mineral density of the mandible is more closely correlated with the femoral neck than the spine, this might be considered the preferred measurement site because it may more accurately reflect the mandibular bone density. However, Holahan and colleagues[43] found no association between implant location in the jaw and implant success, indicating that local bone density was not an important factor in obtaining implant osseointegration. Smoking was found to be an important factor in predicting implant success (hazard ratio = 2.6, 95% CI 1.20–5.63; $P = .016$).

Shibli and colleagues[47] described a case report of a woman who developed osteoporosis about 4 years after placement of her implants. Only one of the retrieved implants underwent histologic analysis, but the bone around the implant was normal. Laboratory experiments have demonstrated that estrogens have a profound effect on bone metabolism, but in the clinical situation when osseointegration has become established they have a minor role in determining implant success. In a larger study of implants removed from 7 osteoporotic and 14 control patients,[48] no evidence was found that osteoporosis interfered with implant osseointegration. These implants had been placed before or at the same time as their diagnosis of osteoporosis, and the implants were subsequently removed largely for reasons of mechanical failure. No bone densitometry was performed on the control group. There was no statistically significant difference between the mean bone-to-implant contact area for retrieved implants from patients with and without osteoporosis. This study was retrospective, and other factors such as implant surface topography, the patient's occlusion, and so forth may have been more influential in determining bone-to-implant contact area and implant success.

In a prospective study of 283 consecutive patients, of whom 187 were females,[49] osteoporosis or poor local bone quality was not associated with a greater implant failure rate up to abutment connection. No statistically significant conclusions were possible, owing the low number of implant failures (14 of 720), although women receiving hormone replacement therapy had a tendency toward a higher implant failure rate. It is highly likely that modern implant surface treatments (such as anodic oxidation, acid etching, and titanium plasma spraying) overcome any minor effects on osseointegration resulting from osteoporosis. The precise mechanisms of early osseointegration are little understood, but the roughness and the composition of the implant surface are important determinants in the rate of osseointegration. Even where studies draw on databases of implants of one particular manufacturer's type, the dentist's choice of implant length and diameter are more important in determining implant loss.[50] Implant studies usually have a very low failure rate, and most studies do not have sufficient statistical power to detect a significant effect of systemic osteoporosis on failure rate.[49] A study involving 399 patients was unable to show any effect of osteoporosis on implant failure, but indicated that other factors (eg, smoking and poor local bone quality) are more important.[51]

In those with osteoporosis, a healing period of 6 months for mandibular implants has been recommended. Even those investigators who describe successful implant osseointegration in these patients recommend a longer healing period or hyperbaric oxygen,[52] but there is little clinical evidence to support this. Given the high prevalence of osteoporosis among older women, it is fortunate that it has a negligible effect on the success rate of implants. In the United States, about 14% of older women older than 50 years have either lumbar spine or femoral neck osteoporosis, and at age 70 years the prevalence increases dramatically.[53] Many implants are successfully placed in this age group, many of whom are unaware that they have osteoporosis. Age and osteoporosis are not therefore contraindicated for implant treatment.

Becker and colleagues[54] found that measurements of bone quantity and quality in the mandible were better predictors of implant loss than peripheral measurements at the ulna and radius (made using peripheral dual energy X-ray absorptiometry). This finding is not surprising, given the only moderate strength of association between the mandibular bone density and that of the rest of the skeleton (**Table 2**). There was no significant difference between the prevalence of osteoporosis in the sample of those who had lost implants (n = 49) and those who had not (n = 49).

A good quality of bone density in the jaws is important in providing primary implant stability. Most assessments of mandibular bone use the Lekholm and Zarb[55] classification, which is a subjective assessment made using dental panoramic radiographs. In the study by Becker and colleagues,[54] implants placed in mandibular bone of moderate to poor bone quality (bone type 3 and 4) were 3.7 times more likely to fail than sites of good bone quality (bone type 1 and 2), but implant failure is not increased in those patients with osteoporosis, provided primary implant stability can be obtained.

Table 2
Correlation coefficients and *P* values between the bone mineral density at the mandibular body and the forearm, lumbar vertebrae, and femoral neck

	Correlation Coefficient	*P* value
Proximal forearm	0.73	<.001
Femoral neck	0.45	.004
Lumbar vertebrae	0.49	.001

Data from Horner K, Devlin H, Alsop CW, et al. Mandibular bone mineral density as a predictor of skeletal osteoporosis. Br J Radiol 1996;69:1019–25.

Most clinical studies show that implant therapy is a successful treatment in patients with osteoporosis.

Despite the lack of clinical evidence for an effect of osteoporosis on implant success, there is evidence of a complicated linkage between osteoporosis, smoking, and tooth loss. Smoking tobacco is a risk factor for osteoporosis and periodontal disease (**Fig. 2**).

The role of periodontal disease and smoking in tooth loss is well established, and there is evidence that osteoporosis is also a risk factor. The mechanism of how osteoporosis affects tooth loss is unknown, but it is independent of local inflammatory disease.[56]

STUDIES IN OSTEOPOROTIC RATS RECEIVING IMPLANTS

Animal models of osteoporosis have involved surgical removal of the ovaries. Implants were placed at varying times after ovariectomy, and the osseointegration process examined. The results of these studies have shown that there are small histologic differences between ovariectomized and control rats in the osseointegration of implants. Duarte and colleagues[57] showed that estrogen deficiency caused a reduction in bone-to-implant contact in the cancellous bone of ovariectomized rats, but this does not result in implant failure. Ozawa and colleagues[58] showed that ovariectomy in rats impedes the early osseointegration process, but functional bone-implant osseointegration eventually becomes established. The effect of ovariectomy in rats on established implant osseointegration was shown in some studies to cause a reduction in

Ovariectomy in animals provides a model for a human postmenopausal osteoporosis-like condition. In many of these ovariectomy studies, the early osseointegration process of implants is affected, with a reduction in early bone contact with the implant. The menopause has not been observed in clinical studies to affect osseointegration, perhaps because the metabolic changes resulting from ovariectomy are sudden and much more severe than those following the menopause in women.

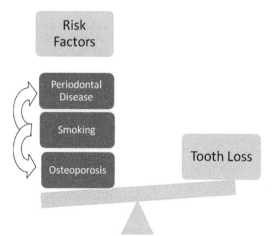

Fig. 2. Risk factors affecting tooth loss. Smoking tobacco is a risk factor for osteoporosis and periodontal disease (*arrows*). Smoking, osteoporosis and periodontal disease are independent risk factors for tooth loss.

bone contact,[59] but Giro and colleagues[60] were unable to show any effect of ovariectomy on the bone contact area of established implants in rats.

SUMMARY

Dentists are in a position to recognize those patients at increased risk of osteoporosis from their clinical risk factors and by observing the thinning and porosity of the inferior mandibular cortex on dental panoramic radiographs. These findings have value in the prediction and prevention of hip fractures,[61] but because they do not provide a 100% accurate diagnosis, it is recommended that dental panoramic radiographs are not taken specifically for the purposes of osteoporosis diagnosis. Because of the radiation exposure, they are to be used when they become available as a result of an investigation for other unrelated conditions. Cone-beam computed tomography imaging has also been shown in a preliminary study[62] to have some promise in detecting mandibular cortical thinning. Because of the radiation dose, it may have a role in the diagnosis of osteoporosis from incidental findings. When patients are suspected of having an increased risk of osteoporosis, it is the author's experience that they value a discussion with the dentist on the merits of further investigation and referral to medical colleagues.

REFERENCES

1. World Health Organization. Assessment of osteoporotic fracture risk and its role in screening for postmenopausal osteoporosis. WHO Technical report series no. 843. Geneva (Switzerland): World Health Organization; 1994.
2. Schuit SC, van der Klift M, Weel AE, et al. Fracture incidence and association with bone mineral density in elderly men and women: the Rotterdam Study. Bone 2004;34:195–202.
3. Gourlay ML, Powers JM, Lui LY, et al. Study of Osteoporotic Fractures Research Group. Clinical performance of osteoporosis risk assessment tools in women aged 67 years and older. Osteoporos Int 2008;19:1175–83.
4. Sedrine WB, Chevallier T, Zegels B, et al. Development and assessment of the osteoporosis index of risk (OSIRIS) to facilitate selection of women for bone densitometry. Gynecol Endocrinol 2002;16:245–50.
5. Karayianni K, Horner K, Mitsea A, et al. Accuracy in osteoporosis diagnosis of a combination of mandibular cortical width measurement on dental panoramic radiographs and a clinical risk index (OSIRIS): the OSTEODENT project. Bone 2007;40:223–9.
6. Roberts M, Yuan J, Graham J, et al. Changes in mandibular cortical width measurements with age in men and women. Osteoporos Int 2011;22:1915–25.
7. Thomas CD, Mayhew PM, Power J, et al. Femoral neck trabecular bone: loss with aging and role in preventing fracture. J Bone Miner Res 2009;24:1808–18.
8. Horner K, Devlin H, Harvey L. Detecting patients with low skeletal bone mass. J Dent 2002;30:171–5.
9. Lee K, Taguchi A, Ishii K, et al. Visual assessment of the mandibular cortex on panoramic radiographs to identify postmenopausal women with low bone mineral densities. Oral Surg Oral Med Oral Pathol Oral Radiol Endod 2005;100:226–31.
10. Damilakis J, Vlasiadis K. Have panoramic indices the power to identify women with low BMD at the axial skeleton? Phys Med 2011;27:39–43.
11. Taguchi A, Tsuda M, Ohtsuka M, et al. Use of dental panoramic radiographs in identifying younger postmenopausal women with osteoporosis. Osteoporos Int 2006;17:387–94.

12. Arifin AZ, Asano A, Taguchi A, et al. Computer-aided system for measuring the mandibular cortical width on dental panoramic radiographs in identifying post-menopausal women with low bone mineral density. Osteoporos Int 2006;17: 753–9.

13. Jonasson G, Alstad T, Vahedi F, et al. Trabecular pattern in the mandible as bone fracture predictor. Oral Surg Oral Med Oral Pathol Oral Radiol Endod 2009;108: e42–51.

14. Devlin H, Allen PD, Graham J, et al. Automated osteoporosis risk assessment by dentists: a new pathway to diagnosis. Bone 2007;40:835–42.

15. Pilgram TK, Hildebolt CF, Dotson M, et al. Relationships between clinical attachment level and spine and hip bone mineral density: data from healthy post-menopausal women. J Periodontol 2002;73:298–301.

16. Renvert S, Berglund J, Persson RE, et al. Osteoporosis and periodontitis in older subjects participating in the Swedish Survey on Aging and Care (SNC-Blekinge). Acta Odontol Scand 2011;69:201–7.

17. Phillips H, Ashley FP. The relationship between periodontal disease and a meta-carpal bone index. Br Dent J 1973;134:237–9.

18. Kribbs PJ. Comparison of mandibular bone in normal and osteoporotic women. J Prosthet Dent 1990;63:218–22.

19. von Wowern N, Klausen B, Kollerup G. Osteoporosis: a risk factor in periodontal disease. J Periodontol 1994;65:1134–8.

20. Elders PJ, Habets LL, Netelenbos JC, et al. The relation between periodontitis and systemic bone mass in women between 46 and 55 years of age. J Clin Periodontol 1992;19:492–6.

21. Takaishi Y, Okamoto Y, Ikeo T, et al. Correlations between periodontitis and loss of mandibular bone in relation to systemic bone changes in postmenopausal Japanese women. Osteoporos Int 2005;16:1875–82.

22. Binte Anwar R, Tanaka M, Kohno S, et al. Relationship between porotic changes in alveolar bone and spinal osteoporosis. J Dent Res 2007;86:52–7.

23. Lerner UH. Inflammation-induced bone remodeling in periodontal disease and the influence of post-menopausal osteoporosis. J Dent Res 2006;85:596–607.

24. Gomes-Filho IS, Passos Jde S, Cruz SS, et al. The association between postmenopausal osteoporosis and periodontal disease. J Periodontol 2007;78:1731–40.

25. Famili P, Cauley J, Suzuki JB, et al. Longitudinal study of periodontal disease and edentulism with rates of bone loss in older women. J Periodontol 2005;76:11–5.

26. Inagaki K, Kurosu Y, Kamiya T, et al. Low metacarpal bone density, tooth loss, and periodontal disease in Japanese women. J Dent Res 2001;80:1818–22.

27. Nicopoulou-Karayianni K, Tzoutzoukos P, Mitsea A, et al. Tooth loss and osteoporosis: the Osteodent Study. J Clin Periodontol 2009;36:190–7.

28. Astrom J, Backstrom C, Thidevall G. Tooth loss and hip fractures in the elderly. Journal of Bone and Joint Surgery 1990;72:324–5.

29. Bollen A, Taguchi A, Hujoel P, et al. Number of teeth and residual alveolar ridge height in subjects with a history of self-reported osteoporotic fractures. Osteoporos Int 2004;15:970–4.

30. May H, Reader R, Murphy S, et al. Self-reported tooth loss and bone mineral density in older men and women. Age Ageing 1995;24:217–21.

31. Klemetti E, Vainio P. Effect of bone mineral density in skeleton and mandible on extraction of teeth and clinical alveolar height. J Prosthet Dent 1993;70:21–5.

32. Earnshaw S, Keating N, Hosking D, et al. Tooth counts do not predict bone mineral density in early postmenopausal Caucasian women. Int J Epidemiol 1998;27:479–83.

33. Krall E, Garcia R, Dawson-Hughes B. Increased risk of tooth loss is related to bone loss at the whole body, hip, and spine. Calcif Tissue Int 1996;59:433–7.

34. Yoshihara A, Seida Y, Hanada N, et al. The relationship between bone mineral density and the number of remaining teeth in community-dwelling older adults. J Oral Rehabil 2005;32:735–40.

35. Steele J, O' Sullivan I. Adult dental health survey. Health and Social Care Information Centre, Dental and Eye Care Team. Leeds; 2009. ISBN 978-1-84636-531-7.

36. Bole C, Wactawski-Wende J, Hovey KM, et al. Clinical and community risk models of incident tooth loss in postmenopausal women from the Buffalo Osteo Perio Study. Community Dent Oral Epidemiol 2010;38:487–97.

37. Iwasaki M, Nakamura K, Yoshihara A, et al. Change in bone mineral density and tooth loss in Japanese community-dwelling postmenopausal women: a 5-year cohort study. Bone Miner Metab 2012;30(4):447–53.

38. Taguchi A, Sanada M, Suei Y, et al. Effect of estrogen use on tooth retention, oral bone height, and oral bone porosity in Japanese postmenopausal women. Menopause 2004;11:556–62.

39. Krall EA, Dawson-Hughes B, Hannan MT, et al. Postmenopausal estrogen replacement and tooth retention. Am J Med 1997;102:536–42.

40. Lee HJ, Kim YK, Park JY, et al. Short-term clinical retrospective study of implants in geriatric patients older than 70 years. Oral Surg Oral Med Oral Pathol Oral Radiol Endod 2010;110:442–6.

41. Glauser R, Ree A, Lundgren A, et al. Immediate occlusal loading of Branemark implants applied in various jawbone regions: a prospective, 1-year clinical study. Clin Implant Dent Relat Res 2001;3(4):204–13.

42. Singh J, Hograth AR, Maini PS. Changes in trabecular pattern of the upper end of the femur as an index of osteoporosis. J Bone Joint Surg Am 1970; 52:457–67.

43. Holahan CM, Koka S, Kennel KA, et al. Effect of osteoporotic status on the survival of titanium dental implants. Int J Oral Maxillofac Implants 2008;23:905–10.

44. Friberg B, Ekestubbe A, Mellström D, et al. Brånemark implants and osteoporosis: a clinical exploratory study. Clin Implant Dent Relat Res 2001;3:50–6.

45. August M, Chung K, Chang Y, et al. Influence of estrogen status on endosseous implant osseointegration [Erratum in: J Oral Maxillofac Surg 2002; 60:134]. J Oral Maxillofac Surg 2001;59:1285–9 [discussion: 1290–1].

46. Amorim MA, Takayama L, Jorgetti V, et al. Comparative study of axial and femoral bone mineral density and parameters of mandibular bone quality in patients receiving dental implants. Osteoporos Int 2007;18:703–9.

47. Shibli JA, Aguiar KC, Melo L, et al. Histologic analysis of human peri-implant bone in type 1 osteoporosis. J Oral Implantol 2008a;34:12–6.

48. Shibli JA, Aguiar KC, Melo L, et al. Histological comparison between implants retrieved from patients with and without osteoporosis. Int J Oral Maxillofac Surg 2008b;37:321–7.

49. Alsaadi G, Quirynen M, Michiles K, et al. Impact of local and systemic factors on the incidence of failures up to abutment connection with modified surface oral implants. J Clin Periodontol 2008;35:51–7.

50. Alsaadi G, Quirynen M, Komárek A, et al. Impact of local and systemic factors on the incidence of late oral implant loss. Clin Oral Implants Res 2008;19: 670–6.

51. van Steenberghe D, Jacobs R, Desnyder M, et al. The relative impact of local and endogenous patient-related factors on implant failure up to the abutment stage. Clin Oral Implants Res 2002;13:617–22.

52. Fujimoto T, Niimi A, Nakai H, et al. Osseointegrated implants in a patient with osteoporosis: a case report. Int J Oral Maxillofac Implants 1996;11:539–42.

53. Looker AC, Melton LJ 3rd, Borrud LG, et al. Lumbar spine bone mineral density in US adults: demographic patterns and relationship with femur neck skeletal status. Osteoporos Int 2012;23(4):1351–60.

54. Becker W, Hujoel PP, Becker BE, et al. Osteoporosis and implant failure: an explanatory case-control study. J Periodontol 2000;71:625–31.

55. Lekholm U, Zarb GA. Tissue-integrated prostheses. In: Branemark PI, Zarb GA, Albrektsson T, editors. Osseointegration in clinical dentistry. Chicago: Quintessence Publishing Company, Inc; 1985.

56. Dvorak G, Arnhart C, Heuberer S, et al. Peri-implantitis and late implant failures in postmenopausal women: a cross-sectional study. J Clin Periodontol 2011;38:950–5.

57. Duarte PM, César Neto JB, Gonçalves PF, et al. Estrogen deficiency affects bone healing around titanium implants: a histometric study in rats. Implant Dent 2003;12:340–6.

58. Ozawa S, Ogawa T, Iida K, et al. Ovariectomy hinders the early stage of bone-implant integration: histomorphometric, biomechanical, and molecular analyses. Bone 2002;30:137–43.

59. Cho P, Schneider GB, Krizan K, et al. Examination of the bone-implant interface in experimentally induced osteoporotic bone. Implant Dent 2004;13:79–87.

60. Giro G, Coelho PG, Sales-Pessoa R, et al. Influence of estrogen deficiency on bone around osseointegrated dental implants: an experimental study in the rat jaw model. J Oral Maxillofac Surg 2011;69:1911–8.

61. Horner K, Allen PD, Graham J, et al. The relationship between the OSTEODENT index and hip fracture risk assessment using FRAX®. Oral Surg Oral Med Oral Pathol Oral Radiol Endod 2010;110:243–9.

62. Koh KJ, Kim KA. Utility of the computed tomography indices on cone beam computed tomography images in the diagnosis of osteoporosis in women. Imaging Sci Dent 2011;41:101–6.

Assessing Systemic Disease Risk in a Dental Setting
A Public Health Perspective

Barbara L. Greenberg, MSc, PhD[a],*, Michael Glick, DMD[b]

KEYWORDS

- Systemic disease risk • Disease risk screening • Coronary heart disease • Diabetes
- Hypertension

KEY POINTS

- Screening and monitoring for systemic disease risk in a dental setting are valuable components toward more effective disease prevention and control, and health care delivery. Data suggest that this can be an effective strategy to identify patients at increased risk of disease yet unaware of their increased risk and who may benefit from proven prevention/intervention strategies.
- The involvement of oral health care professionals in strategies to identify individuals at risk for coronary heart disease and diabetes will extend preventive and screening efforts necessary to slow the development of these diseases, and provide a portal for individuals who do not see a physician on a regular basis to enter into the general health care system.
- Oral health care providers could be an additional resource and an essential component of an integrated public health initiative to control these growing epidemics. Conducting chairside disease risk screening among a targeted set of patients who are asymptomatic and not engaged with a primary care provider (ie, males >40 years of age who have not seen a physician in the past 12 months) could lead to timely behavioral intervention or medical treatment.

PREVENTION AND SCREENING

The integration of oral health care providers into strategies to enhance early identification of individuals at risk of developing chronic disease may be a future public health strategy aimed at preventing and controlling the growing chronic disease epidemics. The purpose of disease prevention and control is to identify individuals who have an increased likelihood of developing disease or experiencing increasing disease severity. Successful prevention is predicated on several underlying tenets, the primary one being the need for an integrated approach that incorporates health care

[a] Institutional Research, New Jersey Dental School, 110 Bergen Street, D 741, Newark, NJ 07101, USA; [b] Department of Oral Diagnostic Sciences, School of Dental Medicine, University at Buffalo, 325 Squire Hall, Buffalo, NY 14214-8006, USA
* Corresponding author.
E-mail address: Greenbbl@umdnj.edu

Dent Clin N Am 56 (2012) 863–874
http://dx.doi.org/10.1016/j.cden.2012.07.011
0011-8532/12/$ – see front matter © 2012 Elsevier Inc. All rights reserved.

dental.theclinics.com

professionals across disciplines. The disease should preferably also have well-recognized, modifiable risk factors, and available, simple, safe, and effective screening tools. Furthermore, individuals who could benefit from screening need to be identified and provided access to prevention programs. A new direction for disease prevention embraces identifying and screening for health indicators and social determinants in conjunction with disease risk indicators.[1]

Screening tests are primarily conducted to assess the risk of developing disease among individuals who present with no clinical signs or symptoms of disease. Early identification of individuals at increased disease risk, yet unaware of their increased risk, allows for early entry into the medical system when medical and or behavioral interventions can affect the risk of disease development. Screening can be considered a flagging mechanism to select individuals who may warrant further confirmatory testing. Screening tests are performed to assess the presence or level of well-recognized disease markers or risk factors and are critical components for strategies to prevent and control disease epidemics. Individuals with positive screening tests are referred to the appropriate health care provider for diagnosis or follow-up for disease/risk monitoring. Screening tests can also monitor an individual's disease progression, and control of individual risk factors once a disease diagnosis is made, or the presence of specific risk factors is confirmed.

WHY SCREEN FOR MEDICAL CONDITIONS IN A DENTAL SETTING?

Screening for risk of developing disease can alert patients to potential disease risks or health issues of which they are unaware. On average, 65% to 70% of adults visit the dentist in a given year, 10% to 20% of whom have not seen a physician in the preceding year, suggesting a potential role for oral health care providers in public health strategies to prevent the onset of, or control the severity of diseases of important public health significance.[2–4] Cardiovascular disease (CVD) and diabetes mellitus (DM) are increasingly important public health concerns that meet the fundamental criteria for effective screening. Screening for medical conditions in a dental setting is a novel approach that could be an effective component of a disease prevention/control strategy that integrates health professionals across disciplines. Implementing screening for systemic conditions in a dental setting should be encouraged not only from a public health perspective but also as an approach to provide additional patient information that could affect delivery of oral health care. Recent data suggest a bidirectional relationship between periodontal disease and diabetes, whereby the presence of diabetes associated with poor glucose control is a risk factor for periodontal disease and may even affect the efficacy of periodontal disease treatment, and the presence of periodontal disease may adversely affect glycemic control.[5–11]

An association between CVD and periodontal disease, independent of common risk factors, has been suggested,[12–16] although data on a causative relationship are inconclusive.[16] Regardless of the exact nature of the relationship between the presence of oral disease and CVD, data support screening dental patients for well-recognized indicators of increased risk for developing CVD, such as hypertension, obesity, and cholesterolemia.

BURDEN OF CVD AND DM

Coronary heart disease (CHD), which constitutes 50% of CVD, is the leading cause of death for both men and women in the United States.[17] According to the American Heart Association (AHA), approximately 13 million Americans have symptoms of CHD.[17] As the life expectancy and obesity rate increase in the population, CVD and

DM are becoming increasingly more prevalent, with 80 million people recognized as having some type of CVD and 26 million with DM; 90% to 95% are type 2 diabetes.[18] The age-adjusted prevalence of CHD decreased from 6.5% to 6.0% from 2006 to 2010, most likely because of improved treatment and control of CHD risk factors.[19] Between 1988 and 1994 and 1999 and 2006, there was an increase in prediabetes from 29% to 34%.[18] The prevalence of undiagnosed disease is estimated to be 29% to 71% for CVD (depending on the specific risk factor) and 27% to 53% for DM and prediabetes.[17-24] Associated with the increasing prevalence of these diseases are increasing levels of disability and growing health care expenditures.[17,18] Recent reports suggest disease prevalence and costs will continue to increase.[25,26]

Primary and secondary prevention activities aimed at modifying well-recognized risk factors associated with these diseases (eg, high blood pressure, high cholesterol, and overweight/obesity) have resulted in substantial reductions in disease-specific incidence, morbidity, and mortality. According to the US Preventive Services Task Force Guide to Clinical Preventive Services, the goal of primary prevention (eg, vaccine administration and counseling to encourage healthy behavior) is to prevent disease onset, whereas secondary prevention (eg, screening) is meant to identify and treat those with disease risk factors and is focused on early identification of asymptomatic disease.[27] Dietary modifications and increased physical activity are associated with a 35% to 77% reduction in the incidence of hypertension,[28-32] a 4% to 10% reduction in high cholesterol,[33-38] an 11% to 15% reduction in incidence of CVD,[33] and a 27% reduction in CVD mortality.[34] Longitudinal studies of lifestyle interventions to prevent DM reported a decrease of 50% in DM incidence during the time of the intervention and a sustained decrease of 41% over a 20-year follow-up period.[35]

Data indicate the beneficial effect of fitness and physical activity on CHD-associated risk factors. Maintaining or improving fitness was shown to significantly reduce the risk of developing CHD risk factors during a 6-year period,[39] whereas supervised exercise significantly reduced levels of existing risk factors, including hemoglobin A1c, blood pressure, high-density lipoprotein, low-density lipoprotein, triglycerides, and body mass index over a 12-month period.[40] No studies have evaluated the impact of oral health care professionals engaging in assisting individuals with lifestyle changes, such as encouraging patients to become more physically active and change unhealthy diets; however, dentists may be reluctant to educate and counsel patients about specific conditions, such as obesity, unless these conditions directly affect a patient's oral health.[41]

Among the numerous screening tools for CHD-associated events, the well-validated Framingham Risk Score (FRS), which uses demographic and clinical measurements, is among the most widely used in the United States.[36-38] The FRS estimates the 10-year risk of developing a severe CHD outcome based on demographic, clinical, and laboratory data.[36] The added utility of additional biomarkers, such as C-reactive protein, is moderate at best and not recommended for routine screening for CHD.[42,43] The AHA's "Guideline for Assessment of Cardiovascular Disease in Asymptomatic Individuals" suggests that measurement of C-reactive protein may be useful in asymptomatic men younger than 50 years and women younger than 60 years with an intermediate CHD risk.[44] Recently, the use of a simple and effective screening test for type 2 DM, the hemoglobin A1c test (A1c), was endorsed by an expert panel.[45] Subsequently, a global study demonstrated that hemoglobin A1c levels can be used to estimate average blood glucose levels for most patients with DM.[46] In April 2010, the American Diabetes Association recommended the use of the hemoglobin A1c test for screening and diagnosis of DM in routine clinical practice.[47] A community-based study validating the use of the A1c for diagnosis of DM found the baseline levels of hemoglobin A1c in an adult population were significantly associated with newly diagnosed DM and CVD.[48] An 8-year longitudinal study reported that the risk of developing diabetes increased as A1c levels increased from more than 5.0% to 6.0% to 6.4%.[49] Use of the A1c point-of-care test is a significant step forward in the screening and diagnosing for DM, as, before this, the accepted screening test for DM required the determination of fasting plasma blood glucose levels.

CALLS FOR PREVENTION AND EXPANDED SCREENING FOR CVD AND DM
CVD

In December of 2012 the US Department of Health and Human Services released Healthy People 2020, the comprehensive set of national public health goals and objectives. One of the primary goals states: "Improve cardiovascular health and quality of life through prevention, detection, and treatment of risk factors for heart attack and stroke; early identification and treatment of heart attacks and strokes; and prevention of repeat cardiovascular events."[50]

In 2012, the AHA presented its new Strategic Impact Goals 2010, which are improving cardiovascular health by 20% and decreasing deaths owing to CVD and death by 20% by 2020.[51] To achieve this goal, the AHA recommendations call for prevention of CVD or promotion of cardiovascular health by encouraging the general population to achieve and maintain ideal levels of 7 behaviors and health factors currently used to define cardiovascular health (ie, not smoking; normal blood pressure, blood glucose, and total cholesterol levels; body mass index; physical activity levels; and dietary content).

Several epidemiologic studies report a low prevalence of cardiovascular health metrics and a significantly decreased risk of CVD incidence and mortality in persons presenting with an increased numbers of ideal cardiovascular health metrics.[52–58] Although age-adjusted heart disease mortality rates have declined 27.8% from 1997 to 2007, risk factor burden remains high, and recent time-trend data highlight the need for improved health promotion strategies aimed at encouraging cardiovascular health.[59] Trends from 1988–1994 to 2005–2010 in these cardiovascular health factors indicate that the risk for CVD and CHD mortality was lower among those exhibiting fewer of these risk factors and that the proportion of the population with ideal levels of all 7 factors had not improved and remains low (2.0% in 1988–1994 and 1.2% in 2005–2010).[60]

Further support for the importance of early detection of individuals with modifiable risk factors is highlighted in recent studies assessing the lifetime risk of CVD based on risk profiles during middle age. Individuals with increasing numbers of risk factors at 55 years of age had increased lifetime risk of death from CVD, as well as risk of death from CHD.[61] In another study of early detection and prevention, the lifetime risk of CVD (starting at age 55 and over an average of 14 years) was lowest among individuals who maintained or decreased their blood pressure to normal levels.[62] Data also indicate the beneficial effect of maintaining fitness and physical activity on CVD-associated risk factors. Maintaining or improving fitness was shown to significantly reduce the risk of developing CVD risk factors during a 6-year period,[39] whereas supervised exercise significantly reduced levels of existing risk factors, including A1c, blood pressure, high-density lipoprotein, low-density lipoprotein, triglycerides, hemoglobin A1c, and body mass index over a 12-month period.[40]

DM

As with heart disease, Healthy People 2020 has a primary goal related to DM, "to reduce disease and economic burden of diabetes mellitus and improve the quality of life for all persons who have or are at risk for DM."[49] Among the 16 stated objectives related to this goal, 3 are particularly relevant and highlight the need for expanded strategies to prevent disease onset and control disease severity; they are noted by the objective number in Healthy People 2020. Objective D1 states: "to reduce the number of new case of diagnosed diabetes in the population"; objective D5 states "improve the glycemic control among the population diagnosed with diabetes"; and D8 states "increase the proportion of persons with diagnosed diabetes who have at least one annual dental examination." The role for oral health care professionals as a component of an integrated approach to disease control is highlighted by one of the objectives under the topic of oral health, which states: "increase the proportion of adults who are tested or referred for glycemic control from a dentist or dental hygienist in the past year." In conjunction with the Healthy People 2020 DM goals, the current strategic plan of the American Diabetes Association has an expanded focus on promoting evidence-based prevention and sets a goal to double the percentage of Americans with prediabetes who are aware of their condition and a 10% increase in people who engage in preventive behaviors.

Data suggest that screening all adults for prediabetes and unrecognized diabetes would be cost-effective compared with no screening over a 3-year period with a saving 6% to 12% depending on the screening test used (including hemoglobin A1c, random plasma glucose, and glucose challenge test) and assuming a 70% sensitivity and a cost for false negatives at 10% of total reported cost.[63] A recently completed 10-year diabetes prevention cost-effectiveness study among overweight and obese individuals showed lifestyle intervention to be more cost-effective than treatment with metformin or placebo.[64]

IS THERE A ROLE FOR ORAL HEALTH CARE PROFESSIONALS?

In previous studies, we developed and pilot-tested a CHD and DM screening strategy for use in a dental setting to identify asymptomatic individuals who are at increased risk for developing DM- and CHD-associated events.[3,65] Demographic (age, gender, smoking history) and clinical data (reported history of hypertension, hypercholesterolemia, CHD, heart attack, stroke, angina, medication use for high blood pressure or high cholesterol) were abstracted from National Health and Nutrition Examination Survey (NHANES) 1999-2000 and 2001-2002 surveys.[3] Data on adults 40 to 85 years of age who had not seen a physician in the past 12 months, but had seen a dentist, were used to calculate the FRS for each study subject to determine their 10-year global risk for developing acute CHD events. Among eligible males older than 40 years, 18% had an increased 10-year global risk for a CHD event (>10% risk score), 14% had a moderate, above-average risk score (>10% and <20%), and an additional 4% had a high risk (≥20%). Extrapolating the study algorithm to the 2000 US Census data showed that among males 40 to 85 years old without reported risk factors, who had not seen a physician, but had seen a dentist in the past 12 months, 332,262 had an above-average and 72,625 had a high 10-year CHD risk.[3] Income and medical care are inversely related, suggesting there may be a significant number of low-income people unaware of their increased risk of CHD who could benefit from screening in nontraditional locations, such as dental settings.

We then expanded on our theoretical calculations with the NHANES data to an efficacy study in an inner-city dental school clinic.[65] Calibrated, trained dentists administered a CHD risk screening questionnaire, measured blood pressure, and tested cholesterol, high-density lipoprotein, and hemoglobin A1c using fingerstick blood collected on a convenience sample of New Jersey Dental School adult patients. Eligibility criteria were: 40 years or older; not being told of having any CHD specific risk factors; no reported history of heart attack, stroke, angina, or DM, and no visits to a physician in the past 12 months. Fingerstick blood was used to measure total cholesterol, high-density lipoprotein levels, and A1c levels chairside with validated machines that yield results within 5 to 7 minutes. Clinical measurements and demographic data were used to calculate the FRS. Among the participants, 17% had an increased 10-year CHD risk (FRS >10%); of these, 14.0% (95% confidence interval [CI] = 10.4–17.6) had moderate above-average risk (>10% and <20%), and 2.2% (95% CI= 0.78–5.2) had high risk (≥20%). One-third of males and 5% of females had FRS higher than 10%. A total of 71% had at least one major risk factor of interest. At the time the study was published (2007) the recommended A1c cut point was 7.0%; at that level, only 1 male was found to be at positive for abnormal A1c levels. Using new A1c screen positive cut points set in April 2010 (>5.7%), 21% would have been at increased risk for DM.

Use of dental settings could augment identification of individuals who could benefit from early intervention. A recent preliminary study in Sweden assessed the diagnostic yield of chairside medical screening in a dental setting.[66] In this setting of universal health care, the heart score was used, which identifies individuals who are at an increased risk of dying from a CHD event within 10 years. Among the 6% who were identified as being at increased risk of dying from a CHD event, 50% were subsequently given medical intervention following evaluation by a physician. These data support earlier work showing the efficacy of chairside medical screening in a dental setting and should be corroborated. Another study in an inner city dental school clinic also supports an important role for oral health care professionals in early disease identification. Unrecognized diabetes in dental patients was successfully identified using 2 dental parameters (number of missing teeth [at least 4] and percentage of teeth with deep [≥5 mm] periodontal pockets [at least 26%]); the presence of either dental parameter had a sensitivity of 73% and adding of A1c measurements improved the sensitivity to 92% compared with fasting glucose. Use of A1c alone showed as sensitivity of 75%.[67]

Given the existence of simple, safe, effective, and relatively inexpensive screening methods, the availability of effective means to identity at-risk individuals and the documented benefit of primary and secondary prevention, chairside screening for medical conditions should be an integral component of dental practice. How do we encourage this practice among dentists? In the behavioral research literature, the theories of planned behavior and reasoned action are the most widely researched principles of behavior change.[68] Fundamental to these theories is the premise that intentions predict behaviors.[69–71] Studies among a variety of health care providers, including physicians, nurses, and mental health providers, show that attitudes are among the strongest predictors of intentions.[72–74] Understanding the attitudes and the perceived barriers to this strategy is essential for success.

Data from a national survey among practicing general dentists showed that 90% of the respondents felt it was important for dentists to screen for medical conditions, and most were willing to conduct chairside screening and discuss the results immediately with their patients, and were willing to refer patients to a physician for follow-up care.[75] A national random sample of US general dentists was surveyed by mail with an anonymous 5-point Likert scale (1 = very important/willing; 5 = very unimportant/unwilling) questionnaire. Of 1945 respondents, a response rate 28%, there was a margin of error of less than 3%. Among the respondents (82% male; 86% white; 60% 40–60 years old; 85% practiced for >10 years), most felt it was important for dentists to screen for hypertension (86%), CVD (77%), DM (77%), human immunodeficiency virus (72%), and hepatitis C (69%); and were willing to refer patients to physicians (96%), collect saliva samples (88%), conduct screening that yields immediate results (83%), and collect fingerstick blood (56%). Based on comparisons of calculated mean ranks, insurance coverage was ranked the least important potential barrier, including time, cost, liability, or patient willingness. Surprisingly, although insurance coverage was important, it was not ranked the most important factor by the practitioners when considering incorporating chairside screening into their practice. A question about potential barriers for incorporating chairside screening into their practice revealed that patient willingness was ranked the most important consideration and insurance coverage was the least important. Other studies conducted since have reported that most dentists feel it is important and they are willing to conduct screening for medical conditions that patients are unaware of or to address medical conditions such as obesity.[41] A study from New Zealand reported that almost all general dentists participated in some phase of disease management of patients with DM, although most were less willing to participate in hands-on activities.[76] Preliminary data among a national sample of practicing primary care physicians show that most respondents felt it was important for dentists to screen for CVD, hypertension, and DM and that they would accept patient referrals based on medical screenings conducted in the dental setting.[77]

An equally important question is how do patients feel about screening for medical conditions in a dental setting. Data from a survey among adult patients attending a university-based dental clinic or seen by community dental practitioners indicate that most patients felt chairside medical screening in a dental setting is important and they were willing to participate in such activity.[78] Confidentiality was their most important concern and not being done by a physician was the least important. Most felt it was important for dentists to conduct medical screening (94%); and were willing to have dentists conduct screening for CVD (81%), hypertension (90%), and DM (83%). Most were also willing to have dentists conduct screening that yields immediate results (91%), discuss results during the visit (88%), receive a referral to a physician (89%), provide saliva specimens (88%), provide fingerstick blood (75%), and pay $10 to $20 (69%). Most felt their opinion of the dentist would improve for competence (76%), compassion (76%), knowledge (80%), and professionalism (80%), suggesting that patients felt screening was beneficial.

A recent review found that repeatedly providing CHD risk information to patients increased a patient's perceived risk and intent to start therapy.[79] Another essential element for an effective strategy to control the global epidemic of CHD and DM is an effective mechanism to refer patients for follow-up medical care and to facilitate referral completion.[80,81] These elements, along with identifying mechanisms for practitioner reimbursement, require further consideration and input from all stakeholders to continue moving this strategy forward.

SUMMARY

In recent years, there has been much written advocating for the creation of a health home to facilitate more effective, coordinated evidence-based health care that integrates medicine dentistry and social/environmental factors.[1,82,83] As part of this health home concept, screening and monitoring for systemic disease risk in a dental setting are valuable components for more effective disease prevention and control, and health care delivery. Data suggest that this can be an effective strategy to identify patients at increased risk of disease yet unaware of their increased risk and who may benefit from proven prevention/intervention strategies. Although there are several issues that require additional consideration and research, there is promise that this can be a more widely implemented strategy. Given that heart disease and diabetes pose significant risks to longevity and well-being, global efforts to move this strategy forward may be warranted. Furthermore, the complex relationship of heart disease, diabetes, and oral conditions disease, highlights the importance of medical screening in a dental setting.

According to the World Health Organization, chronic diseases are projected to be the leading causes of disability throughout the world by 2020 and if not successfully prevented and managed, they will become the biggest problem facing the health care system worldwide. Innovative strategies to combat these growing epidemics are clearly warranted. The involvement of oral health care professionals in strategies to identify individuals at risk for CHD and diabetes will extend preventive and screening efforts necessary to slow the development of these diseases, and provide a portal for individuals who do not see a physician on a regular basis to enter into the general health care system. Oral health care providers could be an additional resource and an essential component of an integrated public health initiative to control these growing epidemics. Conducting chairside disease risk screening among a targeted set of patients who are asymptomatic and not engaged with a primary care provider (ie, males >40 years of age who have not seen a physician in the past 12 months) could lead to timely behavioral intervention or medicaltreatment.

REFERENCES

1. Northridge ME, Glick M, Metcalf SS, et al. Public health support for the health home model. Am J Public Health 2011;101(11):1818–20.
2. Centers for Disease Control. Health, United States, 2010 with special feature on death and dying. Trend tables, table 93. Dental visits in the past year by selected characteristics: United States, selected years 1997-2009. Available at: http://www.cdc.gov/nchs/data/hus/hus10.pdf. Accessed April 19, 2012.
3. Glick M, Greenberg BL. The potential role of dentists in identifying patients' risk of experiencing coronary heart disease events. J Am Dent Assoc 2005;136:1541–6.
4. Pollack HA, Metsch LR, Abel S. Dental examinations as an untapped opportunity to provide HIV testing for high-risk individuals. Am J Public Health 2010;100:88–9.
5. Saremi A, Nelson RG, Tulloch-Reid M, et al. Periodontal disease and mortality in type 2 diabetes. Diabetes Care 2005;28:27–32.
6. Taylor GW, Borgnakke WS. Periodontal disease: associations with diabetes, glycemic control and complications. Oral Dis 2008;14:191–203.
7. Tsai C, Hayes C, Taylor GW. Glycemic control of type-2 diabetes and severe periodontal disease in the US adult population. Community Dent Oral Epidemiol 2002;30:182–92.
8. Lamster IB, Lalla E, Borgnakke WS, et al. The relationship between oral health and diabetes mellitus. J Am Dent Assoc 2008;139(Suppl):19S–24S.
9. Ray KK, Seshasa SR, Wijesuriya S, et al. Effect of intensive control of glucose on cardiovascular outcomes and death in patients with diabetes mellitus: a meta-analysis of randomized controlled trials. Lancet 2012;373:1765–72.
10. Lalla E, Cheng B, Lal S, et al. Periodontal changes in children and adolescents with diabetes: a case-control study. Diabetes Care 2006;29:295–9.
11. Morita I, Inagak K, Nakamura F, et al. Relationship between periodontal status and levels of glycated hemoglobin. J Dent Res 2012;9(2):161–6.
12. Mattila KJ, Valle MS, Nieminen MS, et al. Dental infections and coronary atherosclerosis. Atherosclerosis 1993;103:205–11.

13. Mattila KJ, Valtonen VV, Nieminen M, et al. Dental infections and the risk of new coronary events: prospective study of patients with documented coronary artery disease. Clin Infect Dis 1995;20:588–92.
14. Beck JD, Slade G, Offenbacher S. Oral disease, cardiovascular disease, and systemic inflammation. Periodontol 2000;23:110–20.
15. Southerland JH, Moss K, Taylor GW, et al. Periodontitis and diabetes associations with measures of atherosclerosis and CHD. Atherosclerosis 2012;222:196–201.
16. Lockhart PB, Bolger AF, Papapanou PN, et al. Periodontal disease and atherosclerotic vascular disease: does the evidence support an independent association? Circulation 2012;125:2520–44.
17. American Heart Association Writing Group. Heart disease and stroke statistics—2009 update. A report from the American Heart Association Statistics Committee and Stroke Statistics Subcommittee. Circulation 2009;119:e21–181.
18. Centers for Disease Control and Prevention (CDC). National Diabetes Fact Sheet, 2011. Available at: http://www.cdc.gov/diabetes/pubs/pdf/ndfs_2011.pdf. Accessed April 19, 2012.
19. Centers for Disease Control and Prevention. Prevalence of coronary heart disease—United States, 2006-2010. MMWR Morb Mortal Wkly Rep 2012; 60(40):1377–81.
20. Mozumdar A, Liguori G. Persistent increase of prevalence of metabolic syndrome among US adults: NHANES III to NHANES 1999-2006. Diabetes Care 2011;34: 216–9.
21. Cowie CC, Rust KF, Ford ES, et al. Full accounting of diabetes care and prediabetes in the U.S. population in 1988–1994 and 2005-2006. Diabetes Care 2009;32:287–94.
22. Ayanian JZ, Zaslavsky AM, Weissman JS, et al. Undiagnosed hypertension and hypercholesterolemia among uninsured and insured adults in the Third National Health and Nutrition Examination Survey. Am J Public Health 2003; 93:2051–4.
23. Centers for Disease Control and Prevention. Vital signs: prevalence, treatment and control of hypertension—United States, 1999-2002 and 2005-2008. MMWR Morb Mortal Wkly Rep 2011. Available at: http://www.cdc.gov/mmwr/preview/mmwrhtml/mm60e0201a1.htm?s_cid=mm60e0201a1_e&source=govdelivery. Accessed April 12, 2012.
24. Centers for Disease Control and Prevention. Vital Signs: prevalence, treatment and control of high levels of low-density lipoprotein cholesterol- United States, 1999-2002 and 2005-2008. MMWR Morb Mortal Wkly Rep 2011. Available at: http://www.cdc.gov/mmwr/preview/mmwrhtml/mm6004a5.htm. Accessed April 12, 2012.
25. Boyle JP, Thompson TJ, Gregg EW, et al. Projection of the year 2050 burden of diabetes in the US adult population: dynamic modeling of incidence, mortality and prediabetes prevalence. Popul Health Metr 2010;8:29.
26. Centers for Disease Control and Prevention. Division of News and Electronic Media. Number of Americans with diabetes rises to nearly 26 million. More than a third of adults estimated to have diabetes. 2011. Available at: http://www.cdc.gov/media/releases/2011/p0126_diabetes.html. Accessed January 27, 2011.
27. Sox HC, Berwick DM, Berg AO, et al. U.S. Preventive Services Task Force. Guide to clinical preventive services. 2nd edition. U.S. Department of Health and Human Services, Office of Public Health and Science, Office of Disease Prevention and Health Promotion. Available at: http://odphp.osophs.dhhs.gov/pubs/guidecps/PDF/Frontmtr.PDF. Accessed April 24, 2012.

28. He J, Whelton PK, Appel LJ, et al. Long-term effects of weight loss and dietary sodium reduction on incidence of hypertension. Hypertension 2000;35:544–9.

29. He J, Ogden LC, Vupputuri S, et al. Dietary sodium intake and subsequent risk of cardiovascular disease in overweight adults. J Am Med Assoc 1999;282: 2027–34.

30. Whelton SP, Hyre A, Pedersen B, et al. Effect of dietary fiber intake on blood pressure: a meta-analysis of randomized, controlled clinical trials. J Hypertens 2005; 23:475–83.

31. He J, Gu D, Wu X, et al. Effect of soybean protein on blood pressure: a randomized controlled trial. Ann Intern Med 2005;143:1–9.

32. Puglisi MJ, Vaishnav U, Shrestha S, et al. Raisins and additional walking have distinct effects on plasma lipids and inflammatory cytokines. Lipids Health Dis 2008;16:7–14.

33. Bazzano LA, He J, Ogden LG, et al. Dietary fiber intake and reduced risk of coronary heart disease in US men and women. Arch Intern Med 2003;163:1897–904.

34. Bazzano LA, He J, Ogden LG, et al. Fruit and vegetable intake and risk of cardiovascular disease in US adults: the first National Health and Nutrition Examination Survey Epidemiologic follow-up study. Am J Clin Nutr 2002;76:93–9.

35. Li G, Zhang P, Wong J, et al. The long-term effect of lifestyle interventions to prevent diabetes in the China Da Qing diabetes prevention study: a 20-year follow-up study. Lancet 2008;371:1783–9.

36. D'Agostino RB Sr, Grundy S, Sullivan LM, et al. Validation of the Framingham coronary heart disease prediction scores: results of a multiple ethnic group investigation. J Am Med Assoc 2001;286:180–7.

37. Menotti A, Lanti M, Puddu PE, et al. Coronary heart disease incidence in northern and southern European populations: a reanalysis of the seven countries study for Europe coronary risk chart. Heart 2000;84:238–44.

38. Liao Y, McGee DL, Cooper RS, et al. How generalizable are coronary risk prediction models? Comparison of Framingham and two nations' cohorts. Am Heart J 1999;137:837–44.

39. Lee DC, Sui X, Church TS, et al. Changes in fitness and fatness on the development of cardiovascular disease and risk factors. J Am Coll Cardiol 2012;59:665–72.

40. Balducci S, Zamusa S, Nicolucci A, et al. Effect of an intensive exercise intervention strategy on modifiable cardiovascular risk factors in subjects with type 2 diabetes mellitus. Arch Intern Med 2010;170:1794–803.

41. Curran AE, Caplan DJ, Lee JY, et al. Dentists' attitudes about their role in addressing obesity in patients. A national survey. J Am Dent Assoc 2010;14: 1307–16.

42. U.S. Preventive Services Task Force. Using nontraditional risk factors in coronary heart disease risk assessment: U.S. Preventive Services Task Force recommendation statement. Ann Intern Med 2009;151(7):474–82.

43. Wang TJ, Gona P, Larson MG, et al. Multiple biomarkers for the prediction of first major cardiovascular events and death. N Engl J Med 2006;355:2631–9.

44. Greenland P, Alpert JS, Beller GA, et al. 2010 ACCF/AHA Guidelines for assessment of cardiovascular risk in asymptomatic adults. J Am Coll Cardiol 2010;56: http://dx.doi.org/10.1016/jacc2010.09.002.

45. Saudek CD, Herman WH, Sacks DB, et al. A new look at screening and diagnosing diabetes mellitus. J Clin Endocrinol Metab 2008;93:2447–53.

46. Nathan DM, Kuenen J, Borg R, et al. A1c-Derived average glucose study group. Translating the A1c assay into estimated average glucose values. Diabetes Care 2008;31:1473–8.

47. Lu ZX, Walker KZ, O'Dea K, et al. A1c screening and diagnosis of type 2 diabetes in routine clinical practice. Diabetes Care 2010;33:817–9.
48. Selvin E, Steffes MW, Zhu H, et al. Glycated hemoglobin, diabetes and cardiovascular risk in nondiabetic adults. N Engl J Med 2010;362:800–11, 15.
49. Cheng P, Neugaard B, Foulis P, et al. Hemoglobin A1c as a predictor of incident diabetes. Diabetes Care 2011;34:610–5.
50. Department of Health and Human Services. Proposed objectives to Healthy People 2020. 2009. Available at: http://www.healthypeople.gov/2020/topics objectives2020/objectiveslist.aspx?topicid=32. Accessed January 24, 2011.
51. Lloyd-Jones DM, Hong Y, Labarthe D, et al. Defining and setting national goals for cardiovascular health promotion and disease reduction. Circulation 2010; 121:586–613.
52. Bambs C, Kip KE, Dinga A, et al. Low prevalence of "ideal cardiovascular health" in a community-based population. The heart strategies concentrating on risk evaluation (Heart SCORE) study. Circulation 2011;123:850–7.
53. Khot UN, Khot MB, Bajzer CT, et al. Prevalence of conventional risk factors in patients with coronary heart disease. J Am Med Assoc 2003;290:898–904.
54. Greenland P, Knoll MD, Stamler J, et al. Major risk factor as antecedents of fatal and nonfatal coronary heart disease events. J Am Med Assoc 2003;290:891–7.
55. Magnus P, Beaglehole R. The real contribution of the major risk factors to the coronary epidemics: time to end the "only 50%" myth. Arch Intern Med 2001;161:2657–60.
56. Ridker PM, Brown NJ, Vaughan DE, et al. Established and emerging plasma biomarkers in the prediction of first atherothrombotic events. Circulation 2004; 109(25 Suppl 1):1V6–19.
57. Ridker PM, Rifai M, Rose I, et al. Comparison of C-reactive protein and low density lipoprotein cholesterol levels in the prediction of first cardiovascular events. N Engl J Med 2002;347:1557–65.
58. Danesh J, Wheeler JG, Hirschfield GM, et al. C-reactive protein and other circulating markers of inflammation in the prediction of coronary heart disease. N Engl J Med 2004;350:1387–97.
59. Roger VL, Go AS, Lloyd-Jones DM, et al. Heart disease and stroke statistics. Circulation 2011;123:e18–209. http://dx.doi.org/10.1161CIR.0b013e3182009701.
60. Yang Q, Cogswell ME, Flanders WD, et al. Trends in cardiovascular health metrics and associations with all cause CVD mortality among US adults. J Am Med Assoc 2012;307(12): http://dx.doi.org/10.1001/jama.2012.339.
61. Berry JD, Dyer AD, Cai X, et al. Lifetime risks of cardiovascular disease. N Engl J Med 2012;366:321–9.
62. Allen N, Berry JD, Ning H, et al. Impact of blood pressure and blood pressure change during middle age on the remaining lifetime risk for cardiovascular disease. Circulation 2012;125:37–44.
63. Chatterjee R, Narayan KM, Lipscomb J, et al. Screening adults for pre-diabetes and diabetes may be cost saving. Targeted screening is likely to be even more cost effective. Diabetes Care 2010;33:1484–90.
64. The Diabetes Intervention Research Group. The 10-year cost-effectiveness of lifestyle intervention or metformin for diabetes prevention. An intent-to-treat analysis of the DPP/DPPOS. Diabetes Care 2012;35:723–30.
65. Greenberg BL, Glick M, Goodchild J, et al. Screening for cardiovascular risk factors in a dental setting. J Am Dent Assoc 2007;138(6):798–804.
66. Jontell M, Glick M. Oral health care professionals' identification of cardiovascular disease risk among patients in private dental offices in Sweden. J Am Dent Assoc 2009;140:1385–91.

67. Lalla E, Kunzel C, Burkett S, et al. Identification of unrecognized diabetes and prediabetes in a dental setting. J Dent Res 2011;90:855–60.
68. Perkins MB, Jensen PS, Jaccard J, et al. Applying theory-driven approaches to understanding and modifying clinicians' behavior. What do we know? Psychiatr Serv 2007;58:342–8.
69. Limbert C, Lamb R. Doctors' use of clinical guidelines: two applications of Theory of Planned Behaviour. Psychol Health Med 2002;7:301–10.
70. Walker AE, Grimshaw JM, Armstrong EM. Salient beliefs and intension to prescribe antibiotics for patients with a sore throat. Br J Health Psychol 2001;6: 347–60.
71. Edwards HE, Nash RE, Najman JM, et al. Determinants of nurses' intention to administer opioids for pain relief. Nurs Health Sci 2001;3:149–59.
72. Walker A, Watson M, Grimshaw J, et al. Applying the theory of planned behavior to pharmacists' beliefs and intentions about the treatment of vaginal candidiasis with non-prescription medication. Fam Pract 2004;21:670–6.
73. Farris KB, Schopflocher DP. Between intention and behavior: an application of community pharmacies' assessment of pharmaceutical care. Soc Sci Med 1999;49:55–66.
74. Meissen GJ, Mason WC, Gleason DF. Understanding the attitudes and intentions of future professional toward self help. Am J Community Psychol 1991;19: 699–714.
75. Greenberg B, Glick M, Frantsve J, et al. Attitudes on screening for medical conditions by oral health care professionals. J Am Dent Assoc 2010;141:52–62.
76. Forbes K, Murray Thomson W, Kunzel C, et al. Management of patients with diabetes by general dentists in New Zealand. J Periodontol 2008;79:1401–8.
77. Greenberg BL, Kantor ML, Jiang S, et al. Physicians' attitudes about medical screening in a dental setting. J Dent Res 2010;89(Spec Iss B):4931.
78. Greenberg BL, Kantor ML, Jiang SS, et al. Patients' attitudes toward screening for medical conditions in a dental setting. J Public Health Dent 2012;72(1):28–35.
79. Sheridan SL, Viera AJ, Krantz MJ, et al. The effect of giving global coronary risk information to adults. Arch Intern Med 2010;170:230–9.
80. Sutherland D, Hayter M. Structured review: evaluating the effectiveness of nurse case managers in improving health outcomes in three major chronic diseases. J Clin Nurs 2009;18:2978–92.
81. Dietrich AJ, Tobin JN, Cassells A, et al. Telephone care management to improve cancer screening among low-income women. Ann Intern Med 2006;144:563–71.
82. Glick M. A home away from home. J Am Dent Assoc 2009;140:140–2.
83. Glick M. One-stop shopping. J Am Dent Assoc 2007;138(3):282–3.

Concluding Remarks

The health professions continuously consider their future, and the dental profession will be faced with important questions in the next few decades. Advances in material science and development of new surgical procedures provide solutions to clinical problems that were unavailable just a few years ago. Further, the esthetic desires of patients can be met in a fashion that can change a smile and have remarkably positive effects on a person's appearance and self-image.

However, larger societal issues will impact the profession in the future, including provision of services to individuals who have difficulty accessing dental care, the introduction of mid-level providers, oral health care in health care reform, an increased need for oral health care for the elderly, and the position of the dental profession in the context of health care.

Over the next few decades, the patient population seen in dental offices will be aging. By 2030, 1 in 5 Americans will be at least 65 years of age. These individuals will be retaining all or most of their dentition, but will also be living with chronic diseases and will be managed with multiple medications over decades. The challenge is to provide appropriate dental care for these individuals in consideration of their general health status.

The finding that periodontal disease and periodontal inflammation can adversely influence the severity of certain diseases and disorders at distant sites has also changed our thinking about oral health in the context of general health. Studies examining the relationship of periodontal disease to disorders such as adverse pregnancy outcomes, diabetes mellitus, cardiovascular and cerebrovascular disease, and respiratory disease, as well as other less well-developed associations, have been published in the dental and medical literature. This has increased awareness by nondental health care providers of the potential importance of oral disease for patients seen in medical settings. The microbiota associated with periodontal disease have been identified in atheromas from the coronary arteries of patients with cardiovascular disease[1] and periodontal bacteria have been identified as contributing to adverse pregnancy outcomes.[2] The inflammation associated with periodontal disease has been implicated as contributing to poor metabolic control in patients with diabetes mellitus,[3] and periodontal therapy reduces serum levels of C-reactive protein, a risk factor for coronary artery disease.[4]

The possibility that periodontal disease is a risk factor for different chronic diseases represents a new health care linkage. Building on these associations, dental providers can be involved in the identification of patients with a disease who are unaware of their illness,[5] risk factor reduction, and the assessment of patient compliance with their prescribed course of health care. As discussed in this volume, this can include identification/modification of risk factors for multiple diseases, including hypertension, smoking cessation and obesity management, identification of diseases such as diabetes mellitus, osteopenia/osteoporosis, infectious diseases including HIV and hepatitis C, and dermatological disorders.

An approach to incorporating primary health care into dental practice has been proposed[6] (**Fig. 1**). Patient care in the dental office can be divided into 4 components (patient intake, patient evaluation, diagnosis and treatment planning, and delivery of care). Consideration of the patient's general health would occur in all phases, including visual observation (during patient intake), questioning, follow-up, specific measurements

Dent Clin N Am 56 (2012) 875–877
http://dx.doi.org/10.1016/j.cden.2012.07.012
0011-8532/12/$ – see front matter © 2012 Elsevier Inc. All rights reserved.

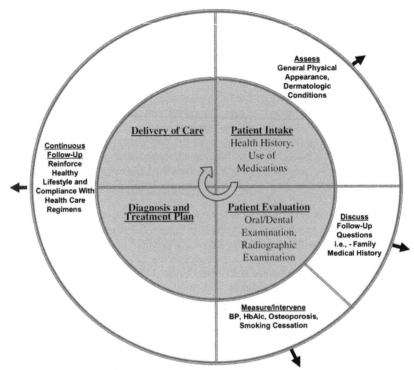

Fig. 1. Incorporation of primary health care activities into the cycle of oral health care. The inner circle is the care provided in a dental office; the outer ring notes specific health care activities that can be incorporated into dental practice. The solid arrows identify points at which referral to other health care providers should occur. (*Adapted from* Lamster IB, Wolf DL. Primary health care assessment and intervention in the dental office. J Periodontal 2008;79(10):1825-32.)

and interventions (during patient evaluation), and continuous, long-term follow-up (during the diagnosis and treatment planning, and provision of care, phases).

Among the most important aspects of this new practice paradigm would be a heightened emphasis on the importance of a healthy lifestyle. As noted in the article on the value of proper nutrition and physical activity by Akabas, Chouinard, and Bernstein, there are 7 modifiable behaviors that have been shown to reduce the risk for cardiovascular disease.[7] These include not smoking, maintaining physical activity, checking blood pressure, blood glucose, and blood lipid profile to assure maintenance in the normal range, weight control, and healthy eating habits. All of these activities are well aligned with the basic tenets of the dental profession; most of these activities would promote health beyond cardiovascular health, have been discussed in contexts by the dental profession, and are addressed in this issue of the *Dental Clinics of North America*.

Dental professionals routinely deliver messages about proper nutrition and reduction of intake of cariogenic (high caloric) foods. The use of fluorides in the municipal water supply and as topical formulations as well as the emphasis on home care and routine professional visits have established a culture of disease avoidance within the dental profession that allows us to more fully embrace a more general emphasis on health promotion and disease prevention.

As noted in a recent editorial that specifically addressed testing for diabetes mellitus in the dental office,[8] many questions remain in this discussion, including issues around the scope of practice, reimbursement, liability, and regulatory issues with the use of point-of-care tests in the dental office. Nevertheless, these are surmountable problems. If adopted, the result will be a more robust dental practice environment and arguably will mean an increase in the provision of dental services, as nondental health care providers refer patients more often, and patients view the dental office as a part of the greater health care system. Fundamental to this change would be that dental professionals would communicate on a regular basis with other members of the health care team, which will also increase these providers' awareness of the oral health care needs of their patients. Benefits would be realized by all involved— patients, providers, and society as a whole.

Ira B. Lamster, DDS, MMSc
Columbia University Mailman School of Public Health
Department of Health Policy & Management
Dean Emeritus
Columbia University College of Dental Medicine
722 West 168th Street
New York, NY 10032

Folarin Odusola, DDS
Department of Dental Medicine
Section of Adult Dentistry
Columbia University College of Dental Medicine
630 West 168th Street
New York, NY 10032

E-mail addresses:
ibl1@columbia.edu (I.B. Lamster)
fo17@columbia.edu (F. Odusola)

REFERENCES

1. Zaremba M, Górska R, Suwalski P, et al. Evaluation of the incidence of periodontitis-associated bacteria in the atherosclerotic plaque of coronary blood vessels. J Periodontol 2007;78(2):322–7.
2. Ikegami A, Chung P, Han YW. Complementation of the fadA mutation in Fusobacterium nucleatum demonstrates that the surface-exposed adhesin promotes cellular invasion and placental colonization. Infect Immun 2009;77(7):3075–9.
3. Correa FO, Gonçalve D, Figueredo CM, et al. Effect of periodontal treatment on metabolic control, systemic inflammation and cytokines in patients with type 2 diabetes. J Clin Periodotol 2010;37(1):53–8.
4. Freitas CO, Gomes-Filho IS, Naves RC, et al. Influence of periodontal therapy on c-reactive protein level: a systemic review and meta-analysis. J Appl Oral Sci 2012;20(1):1–8.
5. Lalla E, Kunzel C, Burkett S, et al. Identification of unrecognized diabetes and pre-diabetes in a dental setting. J Dent Res 2011;90(7):855–60.
6. Lamster IB, Wolf DL. Primary care assessment and intervention in the dental office. J Periodontol 2008;79(10):1825–32.
7. Yang Q, Cogswell ME, Flanders WD, et al. Trends in cardiovascular health metrics and associations with all-cause and CVD mortality among U.S. adults. J Am Med Assoc 2012;307(12):1273–83.
8. Lamster IB, Kunzel C, Lalla E. Diabetes mellitus and oral health care: time for the next step. J Am Dent Assoc 2012;143(3):208–10.

Index

Note: Page numbers of article titles are in **boldface** type.

A

Aesthetics, tobacco stains and, 750–751
Aging of population, in United States, 700, 701, 702
Antihypertensive medications, dysguesia due to, 740
    gingival hyperplasia as side effect of, 738–740
    lichenoid reactions to, 740
    orthostatic hypotension due to, 740
    side effects of, 738–740
    xerostomia and dental caries as side effects of, 738
Asthma, cost of treating, 708
    diagnosis of, projections for, 716, 717
    prevalence of, 707–708, 709, 724

B

Bacteria, oral, and obesity, 836–837
Basal cell carcinoma, 773–775
    clinical presentation of, 774, 775, 776
    pathogenesis of, 773–774
    recurrence of, metastasis factors in, 774–775
Blood pressure, classification of, 733
    effects of medications used during dental procedures, 740–742
    measurement of, 733–734
Blood pressure readings, contraindicating dental care, 737–738
Bupropion, for smoking cessation, 762, 765–766

C

Calories, sources of, among Americans, 792, 793–794
Cancer. See also specific types of carcinoma.
    as chronic condition, 704
    of skin, nonmelanoma, risk factors for, 772–773
        treatment of, 777–778, 779
    oral, diagnosis of, projections for, 723
      prevalence of, 711
      tobacco use and, 752
    persons alive with in United States, 704, 705
    prevalence of, 704–705
    types of, 705, 706
Candidiasis, pseudomembranous, 812, 813

Dent Clin N Am 56 (2012) 879–884
http://dx.doi.org/10.1016/S0011-8532(12)00082-1
0011-8532/12/$ – see front matter © 2012 Elsevier Inc. All rights reserved.

dental.theclinics.com

Cardiovascular disease, burden of, 864–866
    prevention of, and screening for, 866
Caries, and obesity, 837
    and tobacco, 750
    as side effect of antihypertensive medications, 738
    projections for, 720
    smokeless tobacco products and, 750
    untreated, 710, 711
Choose My Plate, 796, 797
Chronic disease(s), diagnosis of, projections for, 725–726
    economic burden of, 701–702
    in United States, 700–701
    prevalence of, 711–724
    preventable, as leading causes of death, 701
    primary care, dental profession and, in United States, **699–730**
Cigarette smoking, and periodontal disease, 748
Combination therapy, for smoking cessation, 767
Coronary heart disease, 864–865

D

Dental care, and hypertensive medications, 737–742
    blood pressure readings contraindicating, 737–738
Dental caries. See *Caries.*
Dental office, assessment and management of patients with diabetes
    mellitus in, **819–829**
Dental profession, primary care, and prevalence of chronic diseases in
    United States, **699–730**
    role of, in obesity, 838–840
Dental setting, assessment of risk of systemic disease in, **863–874**
Diabetes mellitus, and obesity, 840
      obstructive sleep apnea and, 837
    and oral health, 840
      link between, awareness of, 821
    assessment and management of patients with, by dental professionals, 821–825
      in dental office, **819–829**
    burden of, 865–866
    cost of treating, 707
    diagnosis of, projections for, 706–707, 708, 724
    hyperglyceria in, 820
    known, oral evaluation in, 824–825
    oral complications of, 820–821
    periodontal disease and, 820
    prevalence of, 706–707, 708, 724
    prevention of, and screening for, 866–867
    type 2, risk factors for, 822, 823
    types of, 819
    undiagnosed, assessment of patients with, 822–824
Dietary Approaches to Stop Hypertension, caution, controversy, and lack
    of consensus on, 797–798
    diet consumption guidelines, 796
Dysguesia, due to antihypertensive medications, 740

E

Epinephrine, blood pressure effects of, 740–742

G

Gingiva, overgrowth of, drug-induced, 738–740
Gingival hyperplasia, as side effect of antihypertensive medications, 738

H

Hairy tongue, 751, 752
Halitosis, tobacco use and, 751
Head and neck, dermatology of, **771–790**
Heart disease, as leading cause of death, 702
    prevalence of, 703–704, 712, 713, 724
Hepatitis C virus, in dental setting, 815
    in United States, 810–811
    testing recommendations, 812
Human immunodeficiency virus, free rapid test, in dental setting, 813
    in United States, 809–810
    screening in dental setting, 812–815
    screening recommendations, 811–812
    testing recommendations, 812
Hypertension, assessment and importance of, in dental setting, **731–745**
    definition of, 731
    epidemiology of, 733
    importance of, 731, 732
    mechanics of, and treatment strategies for, 734–736
    renin-angiotensin-aldosterone system and, 735–736
    salt/volume overload and, 734–735
    screening for, during dental visits, 737
    sympathetic nervous system and, 736
    treatment of, 733
    white-coat, 734
Hypertensive emergency, symptoms of, 738
Hypertensive medications, and dental care, 737–742

I

Implants, in osteoporosis, clinical studies of, 854–857
Infectious diseases, screening for, in dental setting, **809–818**
Infectobesity, 836–837

L

Leukoplakia, tobacco use and, 753
Lichenoid reactions, due to antihypertensive medications, 740
Lifestyle change, assisting with, role of practitioner in, 804

M

Melanocytic nevi, 785–786
Melanoma, clinical presentation of, 780–781, 782

Melanoma (*continued*)
  incidence of, 778–779
  pathogenesis of, 779
  prevention of, 784
  prognosis in, 783
  risk factors for, 779–780
  treatment of, 781–784
Melanosis, smoker's, 753
Milia, 786–787
My Plate Planner, 796, 797

N

Nicotine gum, 757, 758–759
Nicotine lozenge, 757–763
Nicotine patch, 758, 764–765
Nicotine replacement therapy, 756–768
Nicotine spray, 759–761, 763–764
Nicotinic stomatitis, 753
Non-nicotine replacement therapy, 765
Nonsteroidal anti-inflammatory drugs, blood pressure effects of, 742
Nutrition, and oral health, 792–799
    future directions in, 798–799
    patient's decision matrix for, 804
  and physical activity, in health promotion and disease prevention, **791–808**

O

Obesity, and diabetes, 840
    obstructive sleep apnea and, 837
  and oral bacteria, 836–837
  and oral health, relationship between, 834–835
  and periodontal disease, 835–836
    in children, 836
  and risk of chronic conditions, 709
  caries and, 837
  causes and factors associated with, 832
  cost of treating, 709
  current international statistics in, 832, 833
  impact of, 834
  indicators of, in adults and children, 832
  national epidemic and trends in, in adults, 834
    in children, 833–834
  prevalence of, 709, 718, 719, 724–725
  prevention of, and intervention in, in dental practice, **831–846**
  projections of, 709, 718, 719, 724–725
  role of dental profession and, 838–840
  sleep and, 837
Obstructive sleep apnea, and obesity and diabetes, 837
Oral disease, chronic, 710–711
    prevalence of, 720, 721, 722, 723, 725

Oral health, and obesity, relationship between, 834–835
Oral health care professionals, and systemic disease, 867–869
Oral mucosal lesions, tobacco use and, 752
Orthostatic hypotension, due to antihypertensive medications, 740
Osteoporosis, and periodontal disease, 851
    animal models of, implants and, 857–858
    asseeement of, 847–848
    dental panoramic radiographs in, changes in, 848–850
    implant treatment in, clinical studies of, 854–857
    in dental patients, risk for, identification of, **847–861**
    low body weight and, 850
    risk factors for, 848–854, 857
    studies of, 848, 850, 851–854

P

Patient-centered care, active listening techniques and, 803
    compliance with, 802
    improving oral health outcomes through, 799–804
    issues for health professional, 802–803
    motivational interviewing and, 803–804
Periodontal disease, and obesity, 835–836
    cigarette smoking and, 748
    in children, and obesity, 836
    osteoporosis and, 851
Periodontitis, 710
    diagnosis of, projections for, 721, 722
Pharmacotherapy guide for tobacco cessation, 758–762
Physical activity, and nutrition, in health promotion and disease prevention, **791–808**
    general health benefits of, 799, 800–802
    recommendations for, 799
Primary care, dental profession, and prevalence of chronic diseases in
    United States, **699–730**
Primary care provider, role of, 699

R

Renin-angiotensin-aldosterone system, and hypertension, 735–736

S

Salt/volume overload, and hypertension, 734–735
Sebaceous hyperplasia, 784, 785
Seborrheic keratosis, 784
Skin, functions of, 771
    layers of, 771–772
Skin cancer, nonmelanoma, risk factors for, 772–773
        treatment of, 777–778, 779
Skin lesions, benign, 784–787
Sleep, and obesity, 837
Sleep apnea, obstructive, and obesity and diabetes, 837

Smokeless tobacco products, 748
   caries and, 750
Smoker's melanosis, 753
Snuff dipper's pouch, tobacco use and, 753
Solar lentigo, 785, 786
Squamous cell carcinoma, 775–777
   clinical presentation of, 777
   pathogenesis of, 775–777
   recurrence metastatic potential of, 777
Stomatitis, nicotinic, 753
Stroke, diagnosis of, projections for, 714
   prevalence of, 703, 704, 705, 707, 724
Sympathetic nervous system, and hypertension, 736
Systemic disease, oral health care professionals and, 867–869
   prevention of, and screening for, 863–864
   risk of, assessment of, in dental setting, **863–874**
   screening for, in dental setting, 864, 867–869

T

Therapeutic Lifestyle Changes, diet guidelines, 795, 796
Tobacco, dental caries and, 750
   direct exposure to, 748
Tobacco cessation, barriers to, 768
   in dental office, **747–770**
      assistance with, 753–768
   intervention for, 754–768
   pharmacotherapy guide for, 758–762
   reduction of risks of smoking with, 748
Tobacco stains, aesthetics and, 750–751
Tobacco use, halitosis and, 751
Tooth loss, risk factors affecting, 857

V

Varenicline, for smoking cessation, 766–767
Vasoconstrictors, blood pressure effects of, 740–742
Venous lake, 787

X

Xerostomia, as side effect of antihypertensive medications, 738

United States Postal Service

Statement of Ownership, Management, and Circulation
(All Periodicals Publications Except Requestor Publications)

1. Publication Title	2. Publication Number	3. Filing Date
Dental Clinics of North America	5 6 6 - 4 8 0	9/14/12

4. Issue Frequency	5. Number of Issues Published Annually	6. Annual Subscription Price
Jan, Apr, Jul, Oct	4	$259.00

7. Complete Mailing Address of Known Office of Publication (*Not printer*) (*Street, city, county, state, and ZIP+4®*)

Elsevier Inc.
360 Park Avenue South
New York, NY 10010-1710

Contact Person
Stephen Bushing
Telephone (Include area code)
215-239-3688

8. Complete Mailing Address of Headquarters or General Business Office of Publisher (*Not printer*)

Elsevier Inc., 360 Park Avenue South, New York, NY 10010-1710

9. Full Names and Complete Mailing Addresses of Publisher, Editor, and Managing Editor (*Do not leave blank*)

Publisher (*Name and complete mailing address*)

Kim Murphy, Elsevier, Inc., 1600 John F. Kennedy Blvd. Suite 1800, Philadelphia, PA 19103-2899

Editor (*Name and complete mailing address*)

Yonah Korngold, Elsevier, Inc., 1600 John F. Kennedy Blvd. Suite 1800, Philadelphia, PA 19103-2899

Managing Editor (*Name and complete mailing address*)

Barbara Cohen-Kligerman, Elsevier, Inc., 1600 John F. Kennedy Blvd. Suite 1800, Philadelphia, PA 19103-2899

10. Owner (*Do not leave blank. If the publication is owned by a corporation, give the name and address of the corporation immediately followed by the names and addresses of all stockholders owning or holding 1 percent or more of the total amount of stock. If not owned by a corporation, give the names and addresses of the individual owners. If owned by a partnership or other unincorporated firm, give its name and address as well as those of each individual owner. If the publication is published by a nonprofit organization, give its name and address.*)

Full Name	Complete Mailing Address
Wholly owned subsidiary of	1600 John F. Kennedy Blvd., Ste. 1800
Reed/Elsevier, US holdings	Philadelphia, PA 19103-2899

11. Known Bondholders, Mortgagees, and Other Security Holders Owning or Holding 1 Percent or More of Total Amount of Bonds, Mortgages, or Other Securities. If none, check box □ C None

Full Name	Complete Mailing Address
N/A	

12. Tax Status (*For completion by nonprofit organizations authorized to mail at nonprofit rates*) (*Check one*)
The purpose, function, and nonprofit status of this organization and the exempt status for federal income tax purposes:
□ Has Not Changed During Preceding 12 Months
□ Has Changed During Preceding 12 Months (*Publisher must submit explanation of change with this statement*)

PS Form 3526, September 2007 (Page 1 of 3 (Instructions Page 3)) PSN 7530-01-000-9931 **PRIVACY NOTICE**: See our Privacy policy in www.usps.com

---

13. Publication Title	14. Issue Date for Circulation Data Below
Dental Clinics of North America	July 2012

15. Extent and Nature of Circulation		Average No. Copies Each Issue During Preceding 12 Months	No. Copies of Single Issue Published Nearest to Filing Date
a. Total Number of Copies (*Net press run*)		1054	993
b. Paid Circulation (By Mail and Outside the Mail)	(1) Mailed Outside-County Paid Subscriptions Stated on PS Form 3541. (*Include paid distribution above nominal rate, advertiser's proof copies, and exchange copies*)	505	486
	(2) Mailed In-County Paid Subscriptions Stated on PS Form 3541 (*Include paid distribution above nominal rate, advertiser's proof copies, and exchange copies*)		
	(3) Paid Distribution Outside the Mails Including Sales Through Dealers and Carriers, Street Vendors, Counter Sales, and Other Paid Distribution Outside USPS®	249	306
	(4) Paid Distribution by Other Classes Mailed Through the USPS (e.g. First-Class Mail®)		
c. Total Paid Distribution (Sum of 15b (1), (2), (3), and (4)) ▲		754	792
d. Free or Nominal Rate Distribution (By Mail and Outside the Mail)	(1) Free or Nominal Rate Outside-County Copies included on PS Form 3541	61	63
	(2) Free or Nominal Rate In-County Copies Included on PS Form 3541		
	(3) Free or Nominal Rate Copies Mailed at Other Classes Through the USPS (e.g. First-Class Mail)		
	(4) Free or Nominal Rate Distribution Outside the Mail (Carriers or other means)		
e. Total Free or Nominal Rate Distribution (Sum of 15d (1), (2), (3) and (4)) ▲		61	63
f. Total Distribution (Sum of 15c and 15e) ▲		815	855
g. Copies not Distributed (See instructions to publishers #4 (page #3)) ▲		239	138
h. Total (Sum of 15f and g) ▲		1054	993
i. Percent Paid (15c divided by 15f times 100)		92.52%	92.63%

16. Publication of Statement of Ownership

□ If the publication is a general publication, publication of this statement is required. Will be printed in the **October 2012** issue of this publication. □ Publication not required.

17. Signature and Title of Editor, Publisher, Business Manager, or Owner	Date
Stephen R. Bushing Stephen R. Bushing – Inventory Distribution Coordinator	September 14, 2012

I certify that all information furnished on this form is true and complete. I understand that anyone who furnishes false or misleading information on this form or who omits material or information requested on the form may be subject to criminal sanctions (including fines and imprisonment) and/or civil sanctions (including civil penalties).

PS Form 3526, September 2007 (Page 2 of 3)

Moving?

Make sure your subscription moves with you!

To notify us of your new address, find your **Clinics Account Number** (located on your mailing label above your name), and contact customer service at:

Email: journalscustomerservice-usa@elsevier.com

800-654-2452 (subscribers in the U.S. & Canada)
314-447-8871 (subscribers outside of the U.S. & Canada)

Fax number: 314-447-8029

Elsevier Health Sciences Division
Subscription Customer Service
3251 Riverport Lane
Maryland Heights, MO 63043

*To ensure uninterrupted delivery of your subscription, please notify us at least 4 weeks in advance of move.

Printed and bound by CPI Group (UK) Ltd, Croydon, CR0 4YY

03/10/2024

01040448-0016